The Covid Pandemic and the World's Religions

ALSO AVAILABLE FROM BLOOMSBURY

The Covid Pandemic and the World's Religions

Challenges and Responses

**EDITED BY
GEORGE D. CHRYSSIDES AND
DAN COHN-SHERBOK**

BLOOMSBURY ACADEMIC
LONDON • NEW YORK • OXFORD • NEW DELHI • SYDNEY

BLOOMSBURY ACADEMIC
Bloomsbury Publishing Plc
50 Bedford Square, London, WC1B 3DP, UK
1385 Broadway, New York, NY 10018, USA
29 Earlsfort Terrace, Dublin 2, Ireland

BLOOMSBURY, BLOOMSBURY ACADEMIC and the Diana logo
are trademarks of Bloomsbury Publishing Plc

First published in Great Britain 2023

Cover design and illustration by Annabel Hewitson

A catalogue record for this book is available from the British Library.

Library of Congress Control Number: 2023931567

ISBN: HB: 978-1-3503-4964-3
         PB: 978-1-3503-4963-6
       ePDF: 978-1-3503-4965-0
      eBook: 978-1-3503-4966-7

Typeset by Integra Software Services Pvt. Ltd.
Printed and bound in Great Britain

To find out more about our authors and books visit www.bloomsbury.com
and sign up for our newsletters.

Contents

Notes on contributors

Clare Amos

Until her retirement in 2018 Clare Amos was head of the office for interreligious dialogue and cooperation at the World Council of Churches in Geneva. Prior to taking up this position in 2011 Clare was Director for Theological Education at the Anglican Communion Office in London. A biblical scholar by background, she has taught in Jerusalem, Beirut, Cambridge, London and Kent. She continues to write extensively in the fields of biblical studies, interreligious dialogue and spirituality. Her commentary on the book of Genesis, *Birthpangs and Blessings,* was published in January 2022, and she is currently writing a book exploring the subject of religion and violence. An Anglican Christian, she holds the honorary position of Director of Lay Discipleship in the Diocese in Europe.

Jay Atkinson

Jay Atkinson is a research scholar at Starr King School for the Ministry in Oakland, California, and a visiting scholar at the Graduate Theological Union in Berkeley, California. He served in Unitarian Universalist (UU) parish ministry for thirty-two years until retirement in 2011 and has taught on the adjunct faculties of Starr King and Meadville Lombard Theological School in Chicago (both UU seminaries). His research interests are in UU history and theology, with special focus on the theology and ecclesiology of the proto-unitarian Polish Brethren, who flourished in the Polish-Lithuanian Commonwealth in the years 1560–1660.

George Merchant Ballentyne

George Merchant Ballentyne became a Bahá'í in 1979, in his home city of Glasgow, aged 19. He has worked in the publishing industry and adult education, where he specialized in teaching adults with long-term mental health issues. He was employed by Leicester Council of Faiths as Equality and Diversity Officer (2006–13) and was Voluntary and Community Sector Engagement Manager in the City Mayor's Office at Leicester City Council (2013–21). He has a BA (Hons) from the Open University in English literature and religious studies and an MA from the University of Leicester in Modern Literature: Theory and Practice.

Teipaul Singh Bainiwal

Tejpaul Singh Bainiwal is a PhD Candidate in the Department of Religious Studies at the University of California, Riverside. His research focuses on the Sikh diaspora and how the Sikh faith has been practised in the United States. Tejpaul founded the Sikh American History Project and is the Lead Historian for Stockton Gurdwara. He has written several articles with his most recent publications being: 'Historicizing and preserving the present: The role of music during the Farmers' Protest' and 'Model minority privilege and brown silence: Sikh Americans and the Black Lives Matter movement' (June 2022).

Utsa Bose

Utsa Bose is a postgraduate student in Modern South Asian Studies at the University of Oxford. He completed his undergraduate degree in English at St. Stephen's College, University of Delhi. At Oxford, his research looks at the social space of epidemics in colonial South Asia. He has been interning at the Oxford Centre for Hindu Studies since 2021.

George D. Chryssides

George D. Chryssides is Honorary Research Fellow at York St John University and was Head of Religious Studies at the University of Wolverhampton, where he came into contact with a wide variety of faith communities. He has written extensively on Christianity and on new and minority religions. He was President of the International Society for the Study of New Religions from 2019 to 2022, and is Vice-chair of Inform (Information Network on Religious Movements), based in King's College London. A member of the Church of England, he is a volunteer at Lichfield Cathedral.

Jolene Chu

Jolene Chu is Senior Researcher with the Office of Public Information at the world headquarters of Jehovah's Witnesses. She serves as academic liaison for university-level researchers and institutions with projects in such fields as history, social science, religious studies, medicine, communications, ethics and law. She has studied modern European history and has published on a range of topics regarding Jehovah's Witnesses during the twentieth and twenty-first centuries. Her current research focuses on Jehovah's Witness survivors of the 1994 Genocide of the Tutsi in Rwanda.

Dan Cohn-Sherbok

Dan Cohn-Sherbok is Emeritus Professor of Judaism at the University of Wales. An ordained Reform rabbi, he taught at the University of Kent and was Professor of Judaism at the University of Wales. He is the author and editor of over 100 books dealing with various aspects of the Jewish heritage.

Kumarpal Desai

Kumarpal Desai has acquired an impressive reputation as a writer of inspirational, spiritual and value-enriched literature in India and abroad. He has espoused human values. He is a columnist, professor, former dean of Gujarat University, Professor Emeritus of Jain Vishva Bharati University, Landnun. He has been a columnist of Gujarat Samachar for sixty years. He is a managing trustee of Institute of Jainology. He travels to America, England, Singapore, Antwerp, Hong Kong and Kenya giving lectures on Jainology. He is a trustee, editor and pillar of Gujarati Encyclopaedia. He has written eighty books on Jainism among his 150 books.

Peter Harvey

Peter Harvey is Emeritus Professor of Buddhist Studies, University of Sunderland, and ran an online MA Buddhist Studies from 2002 to his retirement in 2011. He was one of the three founders of the UK Association for Buddhist Studies and edited its journal, *Buddhist Studies Review* 2006–2020. He writes on Buddhist philosophy, ethics and meditation, especially relating to Theravāda Buddhism, with his books including *An Introduction to Buddhism: Teachings, History and Practices* (Cambridge University Press, 1990, 2nd edition 2013) and *An Introduction to Buddhist Ethics: Foundations, Values and Issues* (Cambridge University Press, 2000). He is a teacher of Buddhist meditation in the Samatha Trust tradition.

Usama Hasan

Usama Hasan is currently Director of Al-Quran Society, a UK-based charity devoted to Islamic scholarship. He is a scientist and imam, having been trained in both Islamic theology and the natural sciences: he is Fellow of the Royal Astronomical Society. He has served as an imam, Islamic scholar and Muslim community activist in the UK for nearly forty years, and throughout his adult life. He has translated several Islamic texts into English, and co-authored a dialogue between the three Abrahamic faiths. He has written widely for national and international media.

Vinod Kapashi

Vinod Kapashi is a trustee of the World Congress of Faiths, one of the oldest interfaith organizations in the UK. He was the founder trustee of the Mahavir Foundation and served as president of this trust for twenty-two years. He holds the post of Vice-president in a senior citizens charity called Navjivan Vadil Kendra. He is a spiritual advisor for the Institute of Jainology. He has written twenty-one books on Jain and non-Jain subjects. He has travelled extensively to many countries lecturing on various subjects related to the Jain faith. He received the Honour of OBE for his charitable and religious activities.

Koka Karishma

Koka Kavita Karishma is co-founder of the Ultimate Achievements Academy where she is a Learning Development Mentor, helping to empower individuals by improving learning techniques, communication skills, and self-esteem. Having obtained a BSc degree in Environmental Science and Chemistry, she gained an MSc (Research) in Computational Neuroscience and Molecular Biology from Tata Institute for Fundamental Research, Bangalore. She successfully completed a PhD in Neuroscience at the University of Cambridge on a Scholarship from Cambridge Nehru and British Government Trusts. She is a Fellow of the Cambridge Philosophical Society. Dr Karishma recently founded 'Ba Humata (With Good Mind)' – a project aiming to establish a Global Fellowship among all Zarathushtis.

Taishi Kato

Taishi Kato is a Shinto priest at Hattori Tenjingu Shrine, Osaka, Japan. He was born as the eldest son of a multi-generational family serving their 1000-year-old Shinto shrine. He is committed to introducing Shinto to people all around the world. He participated in The Religions for Peace 10th World Assembly 2019 and the G20 Religion Forum (R20) International Summit of Religious Leaders in Indonesia in 2022 as the representative of Japanese religions. Together with two American collaborators, he produced an illustrated book of Shinto Moments in 2020, which aims to show how religion resonates with the shared human experience.

Oliver Leaman

Oliver Leaman is at the Accademia Ambrosiana and is interested in how rituals in religion respond to changing circumstances. He has taught in the Middle East, Europe and the United States. He has written on Jewish, Islamic and Asian philosophies. His most recent publications are his editions of *The Routledge Handbook of Jewish Ritual and Practice* and *The Routledge Handbook of Islamic Ritual and Practice*, both published in 2022.

Camille Kaminski Lewis

Camille Kaminski Lewis is currently Assistant Professor in the Department of Communication Studies at Furman University in Greenville, South Carolina, USA. She holds a PhD from Indiana University in Rhetorical Studies with a minor in American Studies. Her scholarship focuses on how sectarian religious groups talk their way into the public sphere. She is currently working on a manuscript entitled *Klandamentalism: Dysfunction and Violence in America's Most Romantic Religious Movements*. She attends a Presbyterian church where she is a second soprano in the church choir.

Christopher Lewis

Christopher Lewis is a priest in the Church of England whose most recent post was Dean of Christ Church, Oxford: an institution which contains both an Oxford University College and an Anglican cathedral. He has edited three interfaith books with Dan Cohn-Sherbok: *Beyond Death* (1995), *Sensible Religion* (2014) and *Interfaith Worship and Prayer* (2019), the last having the subtitle 'We must pray together'.

Farhana Mayer

Farhana Mayer studied Arabic and Islamic Studies at the University of Oxford, specialising in Qur'anic Hermeneutics. She was formerly a lecturer at the School of Oriental and African Studies, University of London (2010–12) and the Institute of Ismaili Studies, where she headed the Graduate Programme in Islamic Studies and Humanities (2012–15). She has long been involved in interfaith and Muslim interdenominational dialogue and continues to promote understanding between faiths. She has links with several faith organizations. Her latest publication is a comparative study entitled *An Introduction to Qur'anic Ecology and Resonances with Laudato Si'* (Oxford: Laudato Si' Research Institute, 2023).

Hebron L. Ndlovu

Hebron L. Ndlovu is a bona fide Swazi national and Associate Professor in the Department of Theology and Religious Studies, Faculty of Humanities, University of Eswatini (UNESWA). He received his training in theological and religious studies at the University of Botswana and Swaziland, McCormick Theological Seminary, Trinity College Dublin, and McMaster University. At UNESWA he teaches African Religion, Introducing the Study of Religion, and Religions of the World. His research interests are African sacred monarchies, traditional healing and modernity, interaction of African Religion and Christianity, and multi-religious education. His most recent publications are in the areas of indigenous African Religion, African Christianity and religious education.

Nokuzola Mndende

Nokuzola Mndende is Adjunct Professor in the Department of Sociology and Anthropology at the Nelson Mandela University, South Africa, and formerly lecturer in African Religion at the Universities of Cape Town and Unisa. She is President of Icamagu Spirituality, a national organization based on the revival African Traditional Religion and Spirituality. She is the founder of Icamagu Heritage Institute. She has published extensively on issues relating to African Traditional Religion, Religion and Law in South Africa; gender issues; and Religion in education. She has co-authored eight school books, nineteen peer-reviewed articles in books and in journals and twenty self-published books at Icamagu Heritage Institute as a form of advocacy among the practitioners of the religion.

Wendi Momen

Wendi Momen is a trustee and director of the National Spiritual Assembly of the Bahá'ís of the United Kingdom, a faculty member of the Wilmette Institute (Chicago), Governor Emeritus at the London School of Economics and trustee/treasurer of the Bedford Council of Faiths. She was for many years the multi-faith chaplain at Hinchingbrooke Hospital, Huntingdon. She has written thirteen books on the Bahá'í Faith and has contributed to numerous books and journals. She was awarded an MBE in 2014 for services to the UN Entity for Gender Equality and the Empowerment of Women and to the community in Bedfordshire.

Feargus O'Connor

The minister of Golders Green Unitarians since 2001, Feargus O'Connor trained for the Unitarian ministry at Harris Manchester College Oxford. In 2009 he obtained at the University of Wales Lampeter an MA in Death and Immortality. Since 2006 he has been Honorary Secretary of the World Congress of Faiths (the fourth Unitarian minister in that role) and since 2014 has been Chair of the Animal Interfaith Alliance, of which he is a co-founder. He founded the Clara Barton Disasters Emergency Appeal of the British Red Cross in 2012 and in 2006 the Universal Kinship Appeal of the charity Animal Free Research UK, among whose patrons are Judi Dench and Joanna Lumley.

Shirley Paulson

Shirley Paulson, a Christian Scientist, is the founder and primary contributor for the website, Early Christian Texts: The Bible and Beyond. She was Head of Ecumenical Affairs for the Christian Science Church headquarters from 2010 to 2018, lectured for the Church's Board of Lectureship from 2006 to 2014, and was the Church's liaison with the press and legislature for Illinois from 2002 to 2006. Her academic work is based on studies in theology with a focus on a comparison between Christian extracanonical texts and the work of Christian Science founder, Mary Baker Eddy.

Gary Perkins

Gary Perkins is an independent researcher and author with an interest in the history of Jehovah's Witnesses. One theme underlying his work is that Biblical expectation prepares Witnesses to respond effectively during times of crisis. In 2016 he published *Bible Student Conscientious Objectors in World War One – Britain* and is presently working on a sequel covering Bible Student's responses to war in America during 1917–18. He attends the Carnforth Congregation of Jehovah's Witnesses and is active in his faith.

Anantanand Rambachan

Anantanand Rambachan is Emeritus Professor of Religion at Saint Olaf College, Minnesota. He has published extensively on the Advaita (Non-dual) Vedanta tradition, Hindu ethics, liberation theology and inter-religious dialogue. Rambachan has been involved in interreligious relations and dialogue for over forty years. He is active in the dialogue programmes of the World Council of Churches and the Pontifical Council for Interreligious Dialogue at the Vatican. He serves as President of the Board, Arigatou International NY, a global organization advocating for the rights of children, and as Co-President of Religions for Peace.

Jehangir Sarosh

Jehangir Sarosh, a Zoroastrian originally from India, came to the UK by car and served in the RAF, then ran his own businesses. He is Co-Founder of the European Religious Leaders Council and has served in various capacities on International, European and UK interfaith organizations over the past forty-five years including as the President of RfP Europe 1999–2009. He has presented papers internationally on various subjects including Globalization, Responsibility of Religions, Role of Media and Religions, Freedom of Religion and Belief, and Spiritual Fraternity. His passion is to help religions cooperate for the renovation of the world (the purpose of life according to Zoroastrianism).

Susan Searle

Susan Searle has a Bachelor of Education from the Australian Catholic University and a Master of Theology from the University of Newcastle, Australia. She has been a member of a number of interfaith organization within her community for a number of years. She has presented at CESNUR (Center for Studies on New Religions) conferences in Korea and Israel and other conferences and events in Australia. She is a member of The Mother Church, First Church of Christ, Scientist, Boston, USA, and her local Christian Science branch church, First Church of Christ, Scientist, Penrith NSW, Australia, where she conducts Sunday and Wednesday services and serves on the church board.

Bogodá Seelawimala

The Ven. Bogodá Seelawimala Thera is a Senior Theravada Buddhist monk, ordained in Sri Lanka, and Head of the London Buddhist Vihara (the first Buddhist Monastery to be established in the UK), and Vice-President of the World Buddhist Sangha Council. He obtained BA and MA degrees from the University of Peradeniya, Sri Lanka. He was Buddhist Chaplain at the London Olympics in 2012.

Shaunaka Rishi Das

Shaunaka Rishi Das is Director of the Oxford Centre for Hindu Studies, and serves as Hindu Chaplain to Oxford University. He is a Vaishnava (Hindu) cleric with particular interests in interfaith relations and comparative theology. He served as Chair of the Northern Ireland Interfaith Forum, 1998–2002, and as a Trustee of the Interfaith Network UK, 2002–2004. He founded the ISKCON

Interfaith Commission in 1997 and was Editor of the *ISKCON Communications Journal*, 1993–2006. In 2013 the Indian government appointed him to sit on the International Advisory Council of the Auroville Foundation.

Nikky-Guninder Singh

Nikky-Guninder Kaur Singh is the Chair of the department and Crawford Family Professor of Religion at Colby College in the United States. Her interests focus on poetics and feminist issues. She has published extensively in the field of Sikh Studies. Her most recent books include *Poems from the Guru Granth Sahib* (Harvard University Press, 2022), *The First Sikh: Life and Legacy of Guru Nanak* (Penguin, 2019) and *Of Sacred and Secular Desire: An Anthology of Lyrical Writings from the Punjab* (IB Tauris, 2012). She has lectured widely, and her views have also been aired on television and radio in America, Canada, England, Ireland, Australia, India and Bangladesh.

Koji Suga

Koji Suga is Professor at the Faculty of Shinto Studies at Kokugakuin University. He has been registered as a Shinto priest at the Tochigiken Gokoku Shrine and served for the *kami* of war dead enshrined there on several occasions for more than two decades. He works on faiths and modern society, religions and nationalism, political issues mainly focusing on Shinto and other cases in Japan. He has also researched the relations between religions and technology.

Rowan Williams

Rowan Williams was born in South Wales and studied theology at Cambridge before moving on to research in Russian religious thought at Oxford. He taught at several universities and was Lady Margaret Professor of Divinity at Oxford from 1986 to 1992, when he became Bishop of Monmouth. Having served as Archbishop of Wales from 1999 to 2002, he was Archbishop of Canterbury from 2002 to 2012, and then Master of Magdalene College, Cambridge, from 2013 to 2020. He has now retired to Wales. He is the author of many books on theology and philosophy and has published several collections of poetry.

David J. Zucker

David J. Zucker, a retired Reform rabbi lives in Colorado. His career includes leading congregations in the United States and Great Britain; academia; and for many years Director of Chaplaincy Care at Shalom Park, a senior continuum of care centre. He publishes in a variety of areas: Bible, Chaplaincy and American Jewish literature. His books include *The Torah: An Introduction for Christians and Jews* (Paulist); *The Bible's Prophets: An Introduction for Christians and Jews*; *The Bible's Writings: An Introduction for Christians and Jews* and *American Rabbis: Facts and Fiction* (2 ed.) (Wipf & Stock). See www.DavidJZucker.org. He is a founding member and active participant for over two decades in an Interfaith Chaplains group.

Foreword

by

Rowan Williams

Former Archbishop of Canterbury

Every kind of communal activity was heavily impacted by the Covid pandemic – socializing, sport, education and, of course, the activities of religious communities; this unique collection draws together the questions raised by this experience, and something of the various practical responses of those communities to this dramatic public health crisis – dramatic in a way wholly unfamiliar to 'developed' societies. And it very properly asks what has been learned.

Communities of religious faith have a common concern with both understanding and addressing suffering, and all have to deal with the questions of large-scale and indiscriminate suffering. But they are also concerned with questions about *power*; and perhaps this is something to be kept in mind as we read these reflections. All religious language invites us to think hard about what we mean by human 'power' and challenges the assumption that the ideal human situation is one of unequivocal control over the environment. When we suddenly discover that we cannot after all avoid or manage deep vulnerability, in contradiction to the mythology that modernity has generally disseminated, the blow to social morale is a heavy one. We have to start imagining our humanity in new ways – more honest ways, most people of faith would say. We have to think again about how power might mean not an absolute liberty to dispose of the stuff of this world as we choose but a wisdom about how we confront our limitations and how we deploy the stuff of the world not in a war of competition but in a collaborative attempt to strengthen one another's security. The slogan so popular in the early days of lockdown that 'no-one is safe unless everyone is safe' is a powerful reminder that our safety and the sustainability of our species is something that requires more and more levels of intelligent and compassionate collaboration. Without this – whether it is pandemic disease or environmental disaster that we face – we are going to be increasingly helpless.

But there is another aspect to this challenge. The pandemic mercilessly exposed the different levels of vulnerability experienced by different sorts of community, with those already disadvantaged often bearing the heaviest loads. For many, it was an eye-opener as to the gross inequalities running through supposedly advanced societies, showing clearly how power was gained and perpetuated by some at the expense of others, and how the poorest regularly pay most in our transactions. This is the opposite of the collaborative solidarity we need. And it is painfully difficult to persuade those who enjoy temporary security and prosperity to let go of some of it so as to secure a future for all. How very sluggishly the vaccination process advanced in Africa and other regions deemed less significant in the global economy; how very clear it became that some lives mattered more than others. But the conviction of communities of faith is that human lives cannot be market-rated in this way: what is needed to persuade the powerful of this, and of their share in a common challenge and a common calling?

And for some the requirements of lockdown and masking became an occasion for complaining about how others – especially the state and its experts – were setting out to undermine their freedom; some used the language of faith itself to fuel such protests. There are complex arguments about the rightness of closing places of worship during lockdown, and the traumatic impact of social restrictions on traditions of accompanying the dying and mourning the dead. These essays reflect the sometimes extremely painful debates over the issues; but none of them express the naked individualism that surfaced in some contexts, which vocally resented being made to stand back for the sake of others, or the arrogant pietism that paraded its lack of fear in the face of risk when the deepest risk was to vulnerable others. Power once again, unexamined and unchecked – this time the power of the autonomous individual to choose what they want, irrespective of any shared good or security.

If I have any hopes about learning from these traumatic months and years, it is that we should not forget these questions about human power. If religious communities are to be true to themselves, they are bound to keep challenging the mythology of human arrogance – and, more positively, to remind human beings that to acknowledge dependency and vulnerability is a mark of hope and strength, not panic. These pages return repeatedly to this recognition. They suggest that the process of distilling what is to be learned from the pandemic will need spiritual insight, not just a superficial optimism about doing better next time. There are not many contexts in which what is to be learned can in fact be discussed and processed truthfully and patiently. I hope that our faith traditions will still be able to provide a language and a context where this is possible – because one thing we surely must now recognize is that it is necessary.

Rowan Williams

Preface

The Covid pandemic has been a global crisis. It has caused fear, social disharmony and economic collapse. For nearly two years it has left millions feeling powerless over their lives. In the religious sphere it has brought about enormous change and has challenged basic assumptions about spiritual reality. The aim of this book is to examine how Covid has had an impact on the world's religions. Consisting of twenty-eight chapters from representatives of fourteen of the world's religions around the globe, it provides a panoramic survey of the ways in which religions have responded and adapted to this catastrophe.

The contributors to this volume were asked to address these key questions in assessing how their faith traditions responded to Covid:

1 How does your faith explain why such events occur?
2 How has it affected your religious practices?
3 What changes has it necessitated?
4 What differences might we expect once the pandemic is over?
5 What have we learned from it?

Drawing from widely different perspectives, these voices from around the world have explored in varied ways how the faithful have responded to this crisis. In addition to traditional religions, we have included some that are not so often heard in their own words. We have chosen to include Christian Scientists and Jehovah's Witnesses since the former has attracted a reputation for favouring divine healing in preference to conventional medicine, and Jehovah's Witnesses were vigorously opposed to vaccination at one point in their history. It would be impossible to include all religious traditions, but we have deliberately excluded religious believers who are currently opposed to vaccination, since we did not wish to give a platform to potentially harmful views. They are discussed briefly, however, in the final chapter. It should be mentioned that each author writes in his or her personal capacity rather than as official spokespersons for their faith communities.

Acknowledgements

Most obviously, the editors would like to thank the various contributors to this volume – thirty in all. It would not have been surprising if someone had dropped out or been reluctant to accept our suggestions. We were therefore very pleased that, without exception, everyone delivered their material, and all were extremely cooperative in accepting suggestions for changes. In commissioning such a variety of contributors representing these various religions globally, roughly half were writing in their second language, which is a particularly daunting task, for which they must be congratulated. We are particularly grateful to the former Archbishop of Canterbury, Dr Rowan Williams, for being gracious enough to write the Foreword.

The editorial staff at Bloomsbury are always a pleasure to deal with. We are particularly grateful to Stuart Hay, who dealt with our initial proposal and oversaw the start of the project. Lalle Pursglove, returning from maternity leave, saw the anthology to its conclusion in her usual pleasant and efficient way. Lily McMahon has invariably been helpful throughout the book's preparation.

We should also like to thank our spouses – Margaret Wilkins and Lavinia Cohn-Sherbok – for their support and encouragement throughout. Margaret also deserves our particular gratitude for compiling the index.

Table of acronyms

Acronyms

AN	Anguttara Nikaya
ATR	African Traditional Religion
BAPS	Bochasanwasi Akshar Purushottam Swaminarayan Sanstha
BCE	Before Common Era
CD	Compact Disc
CE	Common Era
CONTRALESA	Congress of Traditional Leaders of South Africa
COP26	Conference of Parties 26
CSR	Corporate Social Responsibility
CSW	Commission on the Status of Women
CZC	Care in the Zoroastrian Community
DRC	Disaster Relief Committees
EC	Executive Committee (I assume this is what is referred to)
FEZANA	Federation of the Zoroastrian Associations of North America
FFP	Filtering Facepiece
G	General Audience
GGS	Guru Granth Sahib
GSR	Green Social Responsibility
JW	Jehovah's Witness
MCBT	Mindfulness Base on Cognitive Therapy
MF	Mahavir Foundation

MP	Member of Parliament
NAWO	National Alliance of Women's Organisations
NHS	National Health Service
NRSV	New Revised Standard Version
NWT	New World Translation
PARI	People's Archive of Rural India
PARZOR	Parsi-Zoroastrian
PCR	Polymerase Chain Reaction
PG	Parental Guidance
PPE	Personal Protective Equipment
PRINCIPLE	Platform Randomised Trial of Treatments in the Community for Epidemic and Pandemic Illnesses
Q	Qur'an
SABC	South African Broadcasting Corporation
SN	Samyutta Nikaya
SOAS	School of African and Oriental Studies
TEC	The Episcopal Church
UK	United Kingdom
WHO	World Health Organization
WZO	World Zoroastrian Organization
ZTFE	Zoroastrian Trust Funds of Europe

1

Covid and religion

Christopher Lewis

How has the Covid pandemic been seen and experienced from the perspective of the very different religions of the world? All religions aim to relate life on earth to a spiritual world, a relationship which sheds light on the lives which we lead, on the love that we show and on the challenges we face. The aim of this chapter is to reflect on the horrific impact of plagues and their double effect: on the advance of science and on the reaction of religion. Religions have made great contributions to the care of the sick; their relationship with the major advances of science has been more varied: occasional rivalry, but in the future, it is to be hoped: a fruitful partnership.

In contrast to Albert Camus' novel *La Peste* ('The Plague'), in which the characters find no meaning in life, religions try to face that life and interpret it for the benefit of the individual, the group, the world. In particular, the question to be asked is: how do we face what seem to be vast and unfathomable threats thrown up by the very world which we have been given to live in? Is this part of some obstacle course which we are challenged (by God) to navigate; is it part of the inevitable growing pains of God's creation; is it an accident which we should have foreseen and coped with; is it a test of our ability to behave as one world rather than as separate rival nations?

These questions are perhaps only faced squarely by religious people when there are natural disasters: eruptions, tsunamis, earthquakes and plagues. Global warming is different; it should be comparatively simple to address because we ought to know both that it is our collective fault and that we have the means to cure it, scientifically if not yet politically. So it would appear that global warming is different in kind to 'natural disasters'. Or is a plague really more like global warming than it is like an earthquake? In other words, should we, at least in modern times, be able to see plagues coming and, having foreseen them, should we not globally and locally be scientifically, socially, politically and religiously well prepared? Bill Gates, who is an international philanthropist and a household name, gave a number of well-publicized warnings, for example, in 2015, concerning plagues, whether beginning 'naturally' or as a 'bioterrorist weapon' (Rogers 2020). Covid began at the end of 2019, and the world cannot be said to have been ready for it; governments and health services were not prepared.

Plagues

Religious thinking has always been exercised by the fact of plagues. Homer's *Iliad*, drawing on an ancient oral tradition and written down in the eighth century BCE, gives an account of the quarrel between Achilles and Agamemnon during the Greek war against the Trojans. Chryseis, the daughter of a priest of the god Apollo, is captured in battle by Agamemnon who refuses to return her. Apollo therefore sends a plague on the Greek army as a punishment, with the result that Agamemnon relents and returns Chryseis to her father.

That tale is a sign of how some Greeks thought about the supernatural long ago: the plague as a sign of the anger of the gods. Such thinking has continued through the ages and is still the pattern for some, although gradually medical science has developed and has shown that the causes are more predictable (and treatable) than was once believed. Hippocrates, born in the fourth century BCE and often known as 'the father of medicine', held that there was no supernatural explanation for illness; he and his followers helped to develop a new discipline separate from philosophy and theology and concentrating on the categories of disease (which included the term 'epidemic') and their treatment.

The history of medicine does not imply that religion is irrelevant. Medicine's advance often involved priest or monk physicians who learned how to treat those who came to them for help. Moses' ancient laws of purification in the Hebrew scriptures may have been learned from medical priests in Egypt during the exile of the people of Israel: a very early example of disease prevention. Such a link between religion, health and healing has continued through the ages. Perhaps the best example has been that of monastic hospitals in medieval times, but many other religious institutions and individuals all over the world have followed a similar path.

Plagues have always been a threat and have had disastrous effects not only on those who have suffered and died, together with their relatives and friends, but also on those who were blamed. The bubonic Black Death in the fourteenth century killed great numbers all over the world, although the estimates are inevitably uncertain: 75–200 million people. The same plague also resulted in many groups being treated as scapegoats: foreigners to the country concerned; Jews, who were said to poison drinking water in wells (Fordham University 1998); beggars; pilgrims; lepers. In Strasbourg in 1349 about 2,000 Jews were massacred as they were seen as the cause of the pandemic. Some religious leaders said that the disease was caused by God; they then said that God was sending the believers to paradise, whereas non-believers were being punished for their lack of belief. There were many other theories concerning the Black Death, including tracing the cause to a conjunction of planets. Whatever the theories, the Black Death returned a number of times, especially in Europe and in the Mediterranean area, right up to the seventeenth century.

Cholera will be mentioned below, but a much more recent pandemic was 'Spanish flu' ('Spanish' was a misnomer) which started at the end of the First World War and led to the deaths of about 50 million people, many of them otherwise healthy young adults. Deaths in that age group demonstrate how difficult it is to study the causes of plagues. In this case, in addition to the ravages of war, it is thought that the stronger immune system of young people probably over-reacted to the particular flu virus, causing death.

It is not surprising that most attention is given internationally to modern epidemics which affect more prosperous countries. For justice properly to be done, the vast threats of diseases such as Ebola and malaria should receive equal treatment to more 'Western' and 'Eastern' plagues. There are countless cases of malaria each year, with over 600,000 deaths (World Health Organization 2022). No fully effective vaccine for malaria yet exists. In 2019, the World Health Organization (set up in 1948) declared the Congo outbreak of Ebola a world health emergency. About the same time, a vaccine was produced, but it has been found hard to distribute in the particular African countries most affected.

Scientific advice concerning pandemics is plentiful, although at times somewhat contradictory. The political reactions to the advice are, however, sometimes hard to understand and may well be ignored as people panic or as rumours and erratic theories spread as to cause and effect. Religious reactions have not always been helpful, for the work of God is sometimes seen as only being done 'directly' and not through the skill of those who research vaccinations or advise governments.

Medical advance

The development of medicine has been a feature of human activity for all recorded history and, no doubt, beyond (Calder 1957). Some progress is lost in the mists of time: quinine (now used against malaria) was a medicine of the Incas in Peru; mould (now the source of penicillin) was applied to septic sores.

Egyptian embalmers learned about the organs of the body and artists learned about anatomy. Doctors from many nations such as China contributed to an understanding of the circulation of blood from about the sixteenth century BCE, although it was not fully understood until William Harvey's work in the seventeenth century CE.

Of more direct relevance to plagues is the fact that by the fifth century CE, Indian doctors had learned that mosquitoes are the carriers of malaria and that rats carry other diseases. In 1403, the Doge of Venice made visitors from the Levant (the eastern Mediterranean area of West Asia) self-isolate for forty days: 'quaranta giorni' hence the word quarantine. Venetians are proud of this fact and took action against Covid in March 2020. There are sightseeing tours advertised as 'The history of quarantine and Venice'!

In 1796, Edward Jenner (a British physician and scientist) created the 'cowpox' or smallpox vaccine, and immunization subsequently became possible for many diseases such as diphtheria and tuberculosis, saving countless lives. In the nineteenth century, the French chemist and microbiologist Louis Pasteur made great discoveries about the causes and prevention of disease, especially concerning the manner in which germs can be killed before they reproduce, much in the way that other living things can be eliminated.

In the 1890s in the United States, a veterinary scientist started studying well-fed hogs which had 'herd immunity' to illness, and that term began to be used in the twentieth century when analysing the build-up of human immunity to various diseases including influenza. Mass vaccination, for example, against measles and polio, began in the middle of the twentieth century. Around that time, there were efforts completely to eradicate smallpox and 'ring vaccination' was used: immunizing everyone in a 'ring' around an infected person in order to prevent outbreaks from spreading.

It is important to note that the use of the results of medical advance is sometimes held up by suspicion on the part of individuals and groups. The psychology of such attitudes is hard to fathom, but people are suspicious of policies which involve personal contact, for they claim 'body autonomy' and they also may say that the kinds of measures which mass vaccination needs in order to be effective are threats to human freedom. Conspiracy theories can spread quickly on social media and may imply sinister motives on the part of those who vaccinate or who limit freedom in order to prevent disease.

Religious development

Religions see, as one of their tasks, the attempt to interpret the world. Why are we like we are and how on earth can we be better both at coping with our own waywardness and also at living in the world which we have been given, with all its complexities? To ask such questions immediately raises another: how do religious thinking and action relate to other disciplines which see themselves as having similar tasks, among them philosophy, politics, sociology and medicine?

The earliest of such disciplines, if it can be called a 'discipline', is magic which was once pervasive in the process of seeking healing and is now less universal, although to say that it is extinct would be a serious exaggeration. It was Keith Thomas who wrote an 800-page book with the title *Religion and the Decline of Magic*, which ends with the wonderful sentence, 'If magic is be defined as the employment of ineffective techniques to allay anxiety when effective ones are not available, then we must recognize that no society will ever be free from it' (Thomas 1978: 800). As the title of the book suggests, religion emerged from an association with magic. On the whole, religion has given a less erratic, more plausible explanation of life on earth, accompanied by better human expression and guidance.

That is not to say that magic should be ignored for it was, after all, the first response of primitive human beings to disease. That many magicians attract the name 'witch-doctors' is significant. Their dealings with the spirit world were no doubt often ineffective (except perhaps in treating mental illness) but they also learned other skills, such as recommending herbs and applying poultices. What is more, like contemporary doctors, they were adept at reassuring the patient, for morale has always been an element in cures; mind and body interact.

Gradually, throughout the world, scientific knowledge developed; magic declined and religion had to alter its understanding of reality in order to take account of scientific progress. There were major dramatic scientific watersheds such as when Galileo, the astronomer and physicist, gave evidence for the theory of Copernican heliocentrism (the earth revolving round the sun and rotating daily), whereas the Roman Catholic Church clung to a geocentric model and opposed Galileo as absurd and heretical. When he was proved to be right, the Church had no option but to alter its views.

That was in the seventeenth century and should be seen as a forerunner of the major shift, at least in Europe, usually called the 'The Age of Enlightenment' and marked by an endorsement of 'reason' and signifying both philosophical and scientific changes as intellectually dominant. Religions had to adjust their views over time, for example (in the nineteenth century), on the evolution of human beings and on the interpretation of ancient manuscripts. More important for our purposes was a general shift in thinking, most pronounced in the West: away from a hierarchical view of life and towards individualism and scepticism. Much of the world changed; not only were there a number of political revolutions, but also industrial and scientific revolutions which led to major cultural transformation.

It is hard to generalize for all religions in this more 'modern' world, but as medical expertise advances together with people's perceptions of healing and health, so religious thinking has adjusted. If a supernatural being (or beings) ultimately oversees all events, what is the meaning of plagues and what is the role of science in prevention and healing? Theodicy, which literally means 'justifying God', is the pursuit of an explanation for why a loving all-knowing deity permits major occurrences which are evil. If these are 'tests of faith', are there not better ways of performing that function?

An analysis of reactions to three pandemics over the last 200 years is helpful in tracing change. Are religion and science at war? Is religion marked by superstition and obscurantism? When medicine produced explanations and effective treatments, how did religion react and adapt?

The first major post-Enlightenment plague was the spread of cholera across the world from India in the 1820s and 1830s. In India itself and elsewhere in Asia, the predominant view of Hindus and Buddhists was that deities, demons and spirits had been offended; Muslims were of the view that Allah's decrees should be endured with patience. Some Christian Churches saw cholera as a divine punishment for human misconduct, the nature of which was at times spelled out: gambling, drunkenness or even opposition to government. Medicine could not offer much by way of convincing alternatives and that led to crowing by the religious: that pestilence baffled scientists or that medicine could only produce 'the impotent boastings of modern science' (Morris 1976: 139). There was a 'half-way house' for some who said that the lives of sinners had predisposed them to disease (Rosenberg 1987: 43) but that view was to be disproved by advances in medical science in the ensuing years.

Those advances should have changed religious views of the Spanish flu of 1918–19. Many faiths, however, still interpreted the pandemic as the will of God or the gods, either as punishment or test. In Africa, there were some who saw the plague as the work of human witches and wizards, resulting in the murder of these magicians (Phillips 2020). Some Christians had taken knowledge of germs to heart, but nevertheless felt that they must not place science 'above' God; they saw the germs as a means by which God could act on sinners.

There were, however, new voices which placed the activity and benefits of medical science alongside God's will. Such thinking continued with subsequent plagues, including Covid. Much prayer changed in character: instead of the request to God to wipe out the plague, it was more a matter of giving inspiration to scientists together with strength to those who suffer and to those who care for them (Galton 1872).

Covid in context

The Covid pandemic has been a matter of worldwide concern for a number of reasons. There are the obvious ones: the sheer number of people closely involved either as casualties or as their relatives and friends; the political difficulties (some would say chaos) experienced as governments have tried to respond too late; the failure to take warnings to heart; the rush to provide vaccinations and other preventive measures, to which is added controversy as to their distribution. Then there is the fact that modern communication in general and social media in particular make both the suffering and the information (e.g. over the distribution of vaccines) more immediate. Those same communications have made it possible rapidly to spread false news and conspiracy theories, for example, the view that vaccines could be the bearer of sinister influences or that to receive a vaccination shows a lack of trust in God.

There are other reasons why Covid is different. For a start, there is the mystery of the source of the original viral transmission to humans in Wuhan in China late in 2019. Then there are its many mutations and the major race to find appropriate immunity to each variant, fronted by countries which have the facilities to manufacture vaccines. How has it spread to be universal and why has it attracted such vast attention and resources? Unlike the disastrous plagues of malaria and Ebola, Covid has had a major effect on wealthy countries and has therefore been the subject of rapid major expenditure.

Religious response to suffering

At the beginning of this chapter, there was mention of Bill Gates as a prophetic figure. One role of religions is to listen to prophets and to make sure that the truth is heard. Governments try to please themselves or their people, but they work with a close horizon; to defend their popularity and perhaps their votes, they concern themselves with the next few years. Religions, with their long-term view of care for people and for the world, can express their views forcefully and give warnings. How much is being spent on research; how will vaccines be distributed fairly, especially to and within poor countries?

It is a particular joy to see science and religion working together. Scientists have discovered their growing need for imaginative ethical thinking and religion has learned of the world's need (and God's support) for good science, so the two have the potential to be in unison.

Another consequence of pandemics is for religions to come together with a common cause. They may sometimes have difficulties in agreeing over beliefs or doctrines, yet there are other aspects of faiths which are much more open to interfaith agreement and activity. One of these is prayer and there is growing experience of people of different faiths meeting together in order to pray about matters of mutual concern. The other is working in support of those who need care and healing. There is much that is inspiring; organizations like the Muslim Edhi Foundation (Winter 2014: 43), the Sikh Hemkunt Foundation or the Christian Leprosy Mission are examples of the innumerable ways in which religions inspire good care of those who suffer.

It is in working to counter suffering in God's world that humanity is called to live out the love that is at the very heart of religion.

References

Calder, R. (1957). *From Magic to Medicine*. London: Rathbone Books.

Fordham University (1998). 'Jewish History Sourcebook: The Black Death and the Jews 1348–1349 CE'. https://sourcebooks.fordham.edu/jewish/1348-jewsblackdeath.asp.

Galton, F. (1872). 'Statistical Inquiries into the Efficacy of Prayer'. Originally in *Fortnightly Review*, 12: 125–35. Reprinted in *International Journal of Epidemiology*, 41 (4), August 2012: 923–8.

Morris, R.J. (1976). *Cholera 1832*. London: Croom Helm.

Phillips, H. (2020). ' '17, '18, '19: Religion and Science in Three Pandemics, 1817, 1918, and 2019'. *Journal of Global History*, 15 (3): 434–43.

Rogers, Paul (2020). 'Coronavirus: Bill Gates Predicted Pandemic in 2015'. *The Mercury News*. 5 March. Accessible online at URL: www.mercurynews.com/2020/03/25/coronavirus-bill-gates-predicted-pandemic-in-2015/.

Rosenberg, C. E. (1987). *The Cholera Years*. Chicago: University of Chicago Press.

Thomas, K. (1978). *Religion and the Decline of Magic*. London: Penguin.

Winter, T. (2014). 'Islam'. In Lewis, C. and Dan Cohn-Sherbok eds., *Sensible Religion*. Farnham, UK: Ashgate: 41–52.

World Health Organization (2022). 'Malaria'. 26 July. Accessible online at URL: https://www.who.int/news-room/fact-sheets/detail/malaria.

2

Pandemics and Jewish responses

Oliver Leaman

Religions are used to the fact that disasters occur and provide means for their followers to make sense of those disasters using the resources of the religion. How adequate those processes may be is a pertinent issue, and for some believers they will be seen as entirely appropriate. For others it is quite the reverse: disasters may be events they cannot cope with using their religion. That is not in itself a critique of religion. We do not criticize medicine as an activity just because there are situations in which it cannot help people, and similarly with religion. We should bear this in mind when looking at some of the reactions in the Jewish world to Covid and the problems it brought along with it.

The problem of evil

Judaism as a religion does not have explicit answers to the problem of evil. The text which most obviously confronts evil is the book of Job, and this ends in ways that are not easy to see as a solution to the problem. Job, we are told, is a good person and yet as a result of a wager the devil has with God on how steadfast he will be when troubles strike him everything goes wrong in his life. His friends come and offer religious platitudes to account for his troubles: he has been bad, disobedient, we just cannot understand divine action – the typical reactions that people with a belief in a benevolent deity tend to display. Yet Job does not feel that any of these responses hits the mark, and he constantly points to the apparent unfairness of what happens in the world. An omnipotent deity should do better, he suggests, and at the very least he gets a response from God to his complaints. It is worth noting that this is far more than most people elicit from God when in similar situations, although the nature of the response is not very helpful in the sense that it relies largely on comparing God with the rest of the contingent world. When God responds to Job He talks about how little human beings understand and how little power they have in contrast with God.

This is not much of an answer, it certainly is not a direct response, and it is far from clear what sense we are supposed to make of it. Bad things happen to many people in the Jewish Bible who seem to deserve better, and ever since prophecy ended Jews have suffered at the hands of their enemies in the human world. Of course, it might be said that unless people could be very bad then we would have no grounds for praising them for avoiding immoral behaviour. Yet when it comes to a disaster that occurs about through natural events, like a plague or epidemic, something that God could presumably prevent, it is not at all clear why He does not do so. To give an example, after the flood God promised never to send another flood and wipe out humanity, yet Covid seemed rather like a flood in its scope and impact on the world. God sent the flood to punish an evil world, we are told. One cannot help wondering if everyone was evil, including the animals, babies, and so on. The idea of bad things happening as punishment is prevalent in many religions, yet while one can see that killing Pharoah's firstborn punishes Pharoah (Exod. 12. 29-30), it hardly seems fair on his son. He did not choose to have the father he had, and as far as we know he was not given to immoral behaviour. The idea that God is behind what happens does ensure a divine role in the world's activities, but is difficult to reconcile with the idea that the deity is fair in what He does. Even Abraham, the friend of God, challenges his friend when He decides to kill the inhabitants of the cities of the plain. He suggests to God that if He is interested in justice then He should consider the fact that there are innocent people there and they will be killed along with those who are more appropriate objects of divine retribution (Gen. 18. 23-33).

This is very much our experience of Covid that the range of people who suffered and sometimes died of the disease was apparently random. Some of them were not wonderful human beings, just ordinary people, while others were blameless mothers and fathers, daughters and sons. Most people who suffered were just ordinary people, neither better nor worse than anyone else. Some took rigorous precautions to avoid getting sick and nonetheless succumbed, while others largely ignored the epidemic and had no problems with it. That is how things work, anything can happen and suddenly lives are changed and brought to what we call an untimely end. Covid brought to the fore what looks like the unfairness in the distribution of rewards and punishments throughout the world, something against which Job so eloquently railed. It is difficult to see any specific Jewish resources or reactions that are unique or different from those of any other religious community. Biblical texts make few and ambivalent references to an afterlife so it is not as though there could be recompense there for the sufferings we undergo in this world. Covid was met with resignation or otherwise by Jews as by other people, and it is worth reflecting on the nature of community here since, as we shall see, this came under some strain and also change during the pandemic.

Jews and communal identity

As with all religions, Jews have very different attitudes to their faith, and indeed to everything. For some Jews their religion defines them in very active and obvious ways. Their days are structured in terms of prayer, eating and drinking certain approved things, living with particular people and dressing in certain ways. They may frequently study Jewish legal texts, their thoughts revolve around their view of their religion and they may accept a particular figure in their community as their leader and authority. Other Jews would not know what a Jewish legal text was and certainly could not study it; they do not knowingly associate with other Jews and never pray or step inside a synagogue. It would be natural, but an error, to distinguish serious Jews from other types, though, since those who do not practise Judaism religiously may nonetheless see it as a significant part of their identity. It is just that they do not see the official rites of the religion as meaningful to them. One of the novel aspects of the pandemic is how new rituals and rites emerged, and as the pandemic wanes it will be interesting to see how they develop or disappear. For example, the decision to close synagogues and communal prayer allowed some Jews who would not in any case go to those institutions to participate and actually become more involved in their religion as a practice. Perhaps they were not members of a synagogue, as most Jews in the United States are not, perhaps they do not know how to pray and were embarrassed to go, perhaps they are unsure of what to do within a communal context. Once services were online they could look and learn and perhaps decide that this was a practice that is meaningful to them and one that they would like to become involved with both during the pandemic and beyond.

New rituals

For some Jews the abandonment of communal prayer and other religious events like weddings and funerals were perceived as disasters and inconceivable events. They saw it as their duty to participate, whatever the secular legal position was, since their communal religious lives are so fundamental to how they see themselves. It was only when the religious authorities themselves forbade such events that many of them reluctantly complied, and often far later than for other parts of the Jewish community. It is not that they give no significance to medical advice or to the demands of the state, but they give priority to their religious duties, as they see them, and they are accustomed to operating in difficult and antagonistic environments. There is a tendency to see such Jews as following a traditional lifestyle, but there is nothing traditional in walking around a hot place like Jerusalem wearing the clothes of a Polish nobleman, and very observant Jews are just as capable of changing their religious behaviour as anyone else. The whole of Jewish law and custom is built around the idea that in different circumstances different things are done, so as with other religions there are plenty of legal ways of explaining and justifying changes in practice, when it becomes necessary to do so. How smooth such changes become varies from group to group, for some it is fairly painless, and for others a big problem, but it is always possible. Using electricity during the Sabbath or festivals may be forbidden and yet if the device is already on and operating, and if it is the only way in which members of the community can safely pray together, then it may be tolerated, even to establish a quorum for prayers where a quorum is required. For Jews for whom the restrictions on Sabbath and holiday activities were never taken very much to heart there was obviously no problem, or so it may seem.

Yet that may be a superficial reaction; there may be no legal problem but there often was a social problem. The phrase 'it's just not the same' was frequently used during the pandemic to describe the effect of doing something which was often done in the past but without others doing it with you in the same physical space. New rituals emerged. For example, vaccination when it became available was often celebrated online as a religious event; a blessing would be recited, people would link it with a festival, candles were lit, and so on. The online community came to take over the physical community, to such an extent that, as with paid employment, many became reluctant to return to doing things with others physically. People often were surprised by this, yet in fact for many years the online lives of people were just as or even more important than their actual lives, so omnipresent has the world wide web become in how we do things and experience the world around us. We tend to see this as the preserve of the young and more secular, but this is not true. Older people have often taken to new technology; it after all is helpful to those for whom physical tasks are perhaps no longer so easy to perform. The religious community is also very much online, on the whole. They tend to restrict the internet to avoid hearing anything of which they may disapprove, such as a woman singing, for example.

Religions and pandemics

The idea of a religious response to Covid is a familiar one, and is behind books like this. There were many discussions during the pandemic on the Jewish approach to it, as well as the approaches of other faiths, and religious figures were often brought in to enunciate what they saw as the main aspects of how their religions see events like that. Cynical observers often detected a depressing sameness in the platitudes that were produced. Life is important, we should promote good health, medical intervention is advisable, we were told, and such remarks are certainly true of Judaism. *Pekuach nefesh*, the preservation of the life of the soul, is a primary duty, and many religious obligations may be suspended or remain unobserved if life is at issue. This is hardly surprising: Judaism did not develop a robust notion of an afterlife until quite late in its history, and it comes via the commentators and not through the scriptures. So this is the only life we have to look forward to and none of the commandments can be carried out if we are not alive. Even those Jews who are persuaded by the rabbinic authorities that an afterlife is waiting for us are supposed to treat their health and their bodies with respect. In cases of illness they do appeal for divine intervention through prayer and other actions, and this was the case in the Covid period also. This is not an attitude prevalent among most Jews in the United States and Israel who are largely secular and unconvinced that God directly intervenes in daily life.

Yet the pandemic with its lockdowns and dramatic changes to everyday life had its familiar effects on those within a religious group, some of whom may have abandoned their links with the religion given the terrible events that went on day after day. Others however reported feeling an increased spirituality, and a spirituality which they felt could be embodied in Judaism. Enforced leisure does after all give people the time and space to evaluate their lives, and perhaps change them. The ability of Judaism, like so many other religions, to change rituals and practices and adapt to the pandemic was experienced by some unaffiliated Jews as a reason to become more involved in their religion, and it is too early as this is being written, in 2022, to speculate on whether they will on the whole revert to their earlier more disengaged attitudes or whether there has been a significant and long-term change. Synagogue members who before the pandemic would attend communal events have not, it seems so far, returned in the same numbers as before, but it is far from clear whether this is due to continuing health concerns about being with other people, something which has also kept workers at home and off public transport. It could be that for some the synagogue attending habit has been broken and they will attend less in future, or hardly at all.

Religions are used to dealing with disasters, they have adapted over the centuries to the terrible things that take place. Plagues and epidemics are hardly new phenomena. Every disaster is of course sui generis, but also reflects the general issue of how we can make sense of a God in our lives who allows such things to happen. Jews have responded in a variety of ways to the Covid event, and there are no indications that it has or will change the religion and those linked with it radically. Religions that have survived for thousands of years are likely to survive a bit longer, Covid or otherwise, and Judaism is no exception. Jews are used to coping with change and may well continue to feel that their culture provides them with helpful resources in this respect.

References

Leaman, Oliver. (ed.) (2022). *The Routledge Handbook of Jewish Ritual and Practice*. Abingdon: Routledge.

Myers, David, Natalie Dohrmann, and Anne Albert. (eds) (2020). *Jewish Quarterly Review, Pandemics and Plagues: Echoes from the Jewish Past*. 25 March 2020. Accessible online at URL: https://katz.sas.upenn.edu/resources/blog/pandemic-and-plague-echoes-jewish-past.

3

Some Jewish perspectives from the United States

David J. Zucker

Seeking explanations

Traditionally Judaism speaks of God creating the world, and being responsible for the orderliness of nature. Prayers describe God as renewing creation daily. The psalms speak of the regular workings of the universe (Pss. 104 and 148). Yet Judaism also understands that there are clear laws of nature which include tsunamis, torrential rains, a dearth of moisture, earthquakes, and the like. Climate change, for example, is deeply affected by human deeds. It is neither God-caused nor divinely preordained. Ps. 33.14-15 reads, 'From God's dwelling place God gazes on all the inhabitants of the earth. God fashions the hearts of them all, observing their deeds.' This statement implies God's omnipotence and omniscience. To be all-powerful does not necessarily mean that God acts all powerfully.

Likewise, to be all-knowing still allows God to self-limit, to choose consciously not to know the future, in order to allow humans free will. In Deuteronomy God tells us, 'I have set before you this day, life and prosperity, death, and adversity … Choose life, if you and your descendants would live' (Deut. 30.15, 19). God wants us to be able to make wise decisions, but if we do not, then we have to live with the consequences of wrongful thinking, action or inaction. Scientific researchers debate the actual origins of Covid-19. We may never know with certainty where and how this pandemic came to be. Whatever those answers, the worldwide spread of this virus can be explained scientifically in terms of human contagion. Covid-19 and its mutating variants are a disease. Judaism does not consider Covid-19 as some form of divine punishment for human misbehaviour. If we choose to follow health guidelines and seek vaccinations, science suggests that we will be more protected; if we fail to do so, we will suffer certain consequences. These are human decisions that we make.

The effect on religious practices

Covid-19 and its variants, and more specifically the fear of its transmission and spread through particles in the air as the result of human breath, have resulted in the suspension of many activities, where before people were in close contact with one another. Under normal conditions in Jewish life, Jews come together to pray, to participate in meetings, to learn, to socialize and to support one another at life-cycle events. In terms of prayer, the most common locale is at a synagogue, whether this is on a daily, or a weekly basis on the Jewish Shabbat (Sabbath) or at various festivals and High Holy Days throughout the year. Because of requirements for masking and social distancing, and then the fear of contagion, most synagogues chose – at least for a period – to suspend in-person religious services.

Judaism is the religion of Jews. Jews, however, are more than just a religion. Jews are a people, a culture, an ethnic group, hence Jews meet as Jews for various reasons, which might be broadly defined as educational, social, religious, philanthropic, political or professional gatherings, to name but a few categories. Because of 'social distancing' and then the fear of contagion, the organizers of many of these meetings, whether secular or religiously connected as in the general religious sphere, chose to suspend in-person public gatherings and replace them with digital alternatives – the world of 'virtual' communication.

What changes has it necessitated

The suspension of regular – dare one say 'normal' – public gatherings resulted in some very creative ways of communicating. Covid-19 brought about a popular digital revolution. Jewish religious as well as thousands of secular organizations adapted and did and do make use of all kinds of virtual formats where oftentimes one can interact or speak with others. Many synagogues outside of the world of Orthodoxy now have both in-person and virtual services available electronically. These hybrid services appear to be a permanent fixture.

The need for social distancing and the real fear of contagion impact life-cycle events. It is commonplace now to utilize virtual technology at funerals.

Likewise, *shiva* services (the post-funeral prayer services) are accessible in a virtual format. In Judaism, a child is bar-mitzvah or bat-mitzvah simply because they have come of age. They may or may not formally choose to lead part of the regular synagogue service and read from the Torah, but simply because they are of age (twelve or thirteen for girls, thirteen for boys), they are counted as adults as part of the prayer quorum. In-person bar-mitzvah and bat-mitzvah services (the former for boys and the latter for girls) are often limited to immediate family, and possibly close relatives and friends, although additionally accessible via virtual technology. In some cases, weddings were postponed in the hope that the social distancing requirements will or would not be required.

The various streams or branches in Judaism – Reconstructionist-Reform-Conservative-Orthodox – approached the 'in-person' issue differently. Generally Reconstructionist and Reform congregations opted for virtual technology in the form of electronic transmission of weekly Shabbat, Festival and High Holy Day services through the strategic use of cameras in the sanctuary. Initially clergy led the services but in the absence of actual congregants, with congregants present virtually. Numerous synagogues still encourage, but do not require masking and social distancing.

Many Conservative congregations followed a similar kind of regimen. In the Orthodox community there was a variety of responses. In the Ultra-Orthodox Hasidic (Haredi) community certainly some chose to ignore the government's proposed guidelines. They did meet in person and ignored social distancing. The result was widespread infections. In other situations, there was an attempt to limit the 'in-person' prayer services to ten men (the required minimum number for a *minyan*) or perhaps an even larger number depending on space, whilst practising social distancing. In other congregations, weather permitting, people met to pray outside, near the synagogue. In the more mainstream Orthodox communities, like the other branches of Judaism, synagogues were initially closed for several months beginning in March 2020. Opening was a slow process (again true for all branches). A number started to open with a small weekday prayer service (*minyan*) so long as people were vaccinated or had boosters, were masked and socially distanced.

In time, the Orthodox synagogues opened for daily, weekly Shabbat as well as Festival, and High Holy Day services – again like the other branches in Judaism – with the stipulations of full vaccination and boosters, as well as mask, social distancing requirements and other safety measures. Weekday services in some cases were streamed. Not atypical was the example of an Orthodox synagogue which installed a heavy plastic see-through enclosure around the lectern in the Sanctuary so the Cantor could sing freely without a mask. The Torah scroll was taken from the ark directly to the reading desk and read there. It was not processed through the congregation. Individual blessings (*aliyot*) were taken from seats. There were sign-up requirements to attend any of the services. With some variations such as allowing people to come up to the Torah to recite blessings (*aliyot*), their procedure was like Reconstructionist, Reform and Conservative congregations. In some cases for synagogues, for daily but not Shabbat or festivals, the use of virtual technology allowed people to recite either part of the prayers or the Torah blessings (*aliyot*) from their homes. Synagogues across the board made some modifications to the service length, primarily on Shabbat, Festival and especially the High Holy Day services. Likewise, oftentimes the rabbi's sermon was more limited in time. In some synagogues the rabbi videotaped the sermon and sent it out electronically before Shabbat or the Holy Day. During the first year of Covid-19, no one really knew fully how the pandemic would play out. Being in a building for an inordinate length of time – especially with a mask – was difficult and, at least at that time, was unwise.

In terms of the High Holy Days, many non-Orthodox synagogues decided to use virtual technology, to stream their services in 2020 and, again, in 2021. In 2021 and 2022, there were both in-person and virtual services. Many congregants, certainly of a more mature age, appeared fearful of contagion if they attended services in person.

No doubt, depending on the synagogue's traditions, or the rabbi's definition of what is or is not permitted on Shabbat or festivals, in terms of electronic usage, congregations differ in their approach to these questions. Switching on a computer before the Shabbat or festival begins is one approach, but generally in the more observant world, this would be violating the spirit of the tradition. Switching on a computer on Shabbat or a festival would be regarded as in a similar category to pressing a key to join a YouTube streamed service. This interpretation of electronic usage is based on Exod. 35.3, 'You shall kindle no fire throughout your settlements on the sabbath day.'

Universally, a bar-mitzvah or bat-mitzvah with the availability of streaming (though in more observant or traditionally oriented congregations not on Shabbat) is understood as the new norm. The child does what he or she does, whether it is reading certain prayers, or from the Torah. Given that the pandemic is clearly a multiple-year phenomenon, there will not be a 'now we can have the "real" service, albeit postponed' because there is a set liturgical calendar for each year. That service, streamed or not, is the only service.

Across the board, in terms of synagogue meetings, congregations quickly adjusted to virtual activities. Some religious school classes had in-person mask requirements; others were taught online. Online Jewish education is flourishing. Further, by recording learning sessions and then making them available, people can access these programmes later; they need not be there in person to receive this instruction. The pandemic brought new opportunities, not only by way of education. Synagogue and secular boards have been able to invite older and younger members to participate through virtual technology, including parents of young children who otherwise would not be able to get away in the evening because of parental duties.

For all the benefits of virtual technology, there are downsides as well. There is no way that the speaker can make direct eye contact with virtual technology participants. Likewise, there is no way to coordinate unmuted community chanting or singing, because even split-second differences result in a cacophonous sound. Virtual technology accomplishes certain ends; however, it cannot replicate the positive social aspects and benefits of a *Kiddush* or *Oneg* (in-person, human social connection, with refreshments following a service). People need that kind of direct human-contact experience. How to bring that about safely and to achieve pre-pandemic numbers is an ongoing challenge.

An Orthodox congregational leader in Queens, New York (who was ordained at the centrist/mainstream Rabbi Isaac Elchanan Theological Seminary – Yeshiva University) Rabbi Judah Kerbel, writes that 'an element of synagogue life that is even more difficult to create virtually than prayer and learning [is] the social-communal relationships generated by synagogue participation' (Kerbel 2021). He quotes engagement expert Ron Wolfson, who writes that synagogue 'is not about programs. It's not about branding, labels, logos, clever titles, websites or smartphone apps. It's not even about institutions. *It's about relationships*' (Wolfson 2013: 2–3; quoted in Kerbel, italics original). Kerbel continues, 'While the primary, expressed purpose of synagogue is our relationship with God, there is a lot of truth to the notion that we come to synagogue to connect with other people.'

A whole different aspect in terms of the pandemic and how it has necessitated changes are the experiences that impacted Jewish chaplains. Like their fellow chaplains of other religious groupings, Jewish chaplains faced unprecedented questions: how, given the ubiquitous literal presence of Covid-19 among patients, could the chaplain be of help as a 'pastoral presence', whether in hospitals, long-term care facilities, hospices or prisons? How does one interact with patients, residents, clients or prisoners when due to health regulations one cannot enter the room, or one has to be masked and gowned and it is literally forbidden to 'reach out and touch' someone? How best to be a pastoral presence and interact with families who, again because of Covid-19 restrictions, could not enter the facility, much less see their loved one in person? How to support the medical staff (doctors, nurses and auxiliary staff) who are themselves feeling the increased pressures of a near-capacity census? Or how to best be a pastoral presence when there are tensions due to turnovers in staffing (other institutions offering greater remuneration for services). How does one stay safe and healthy physically, emotionally and spiritually where, oftentimes by definition, one is working in a high-risk environment?

Changes after the pandemic

There seems to be universal agreement among the religious spectrum that hybrid programming (in-person, with or without masking and social distancing) using virtual technology is the 'new normal'. Without question, larger congregations with more robust budgeting will be able to offer more sophisticated programming and access to religious services. Nonetheless, there will be limitations in terms of sound and visual quality. Religious and lay leaders no doubt will have to adjust to learning how to 'speak' to a camera, even as they will also need to adjust to speaking simultaneously to their live congregation or audience, depending on whether this is a religious service or a secular programme. No doubt, in the future many meetings will feature both in-person and virtual options. It is clear that many synagogues (as is true with other religions) are finding that there is a very slow 'return to the pews'. Attendances are considerably lower than pre-pandemic times. There has been an economic aspect to the Pandemic which directly affects the bottom line of institutional budgets. Synagogues with large buildings may well find ways to share space with other organizations.

In April 2022, an essay raised some of the questions that will need to be addressed. It was titled, 'Lessons from the Pandemic for Congregations and Community Organizing / Lecciones de la Pandemia para las Congregaciones y el Trabajo Organizador Comunitario.' It noted that 'at this point, it is too early to say definitively what the lasting effects of the pandemic will be, but a number of significant, even existential, questions loom' (Fleming and James-Saadiya 2022). These questions will try to address what will be the lasting effects for the emotional, spiritual and physical health of clergy and lay members. Will congregants who used to attend worship services on a weekly or regular basis return to their pre-pandemic practices? What will be the long-term financial implications for congregations that have lost members and financial resources? Will congregations need to close? What will fill the spiritual void if congregations do not remain viable? Are faith communities prepared to respond to that impact and ongoing need?

What have we learned?

Life changes. We may not be comfortable, at least in the short run, with making the kinds of modifications that will be required, but they will be necessary in the future hybrid virtual technology world in which we shall live. Technology developed out of necessity in the pandemic world has also brought some positive aspects in its wake. People who were unable to attend religious services or other kinds of programming because of health issues, distance or climatic conditions now through virtual technology can be 'active' participants. Again, organizations which are better funded will be able to do more sophisticated programming. Regardless of this, through virtual technology there will be both more equal and more widespread opportunities and resources available to people who up till now may have been excluded or marginalized. The question how one can establish and maintain meaningful relationship-based communities will define the success of the 'new normal'.

References

Fleming, Joe, and Rashida James-Saadiya (2022). 'Lessons from the Pandemic for Congregations and Community Organizing / Lecciones de la Pandemia para las Congregaciones y el Trabajo Organizador Comunitario'. *Faith in Action.* 25 April. Accessible online at URL: https://faithinaction.org/our-stories.

Kerbel, Judah (2021). 'The Synagogue after Corona: From Crisis to Opportunity'. *Lehrhaus.* 4 January. Accessible online at URL: https://thelehrhaus.com/coronavirus/the-synagogue-after-corona-from-crisis-to-opportunity/#_edn3.

Wolfson, Ron (2013). *Relational Judaism: Using the Power of Relationships to Transform the Jewish Community.* Woodstock: Jewish Lights Publishing.

4

Covid, Communion and Christianity

Clare Amos

My husband, Alan Amos, who is an Anglican priest, writes poetry. I can be his harshest critic! However the Covid pandemic, especially in its first few months, led to Alan's poetic muse working overtime, and he composed several pieces that reached a wide and appreciative audience.

Perhaps my own favourite was written on the first 'Good Friday' of the pandemic period. Holy Trinity, the Anglican Church in Geneva with which we have been associated during the last decade, had moved its services online. Alan and I were involved in helping to design and present the online services for Holy Week and Easter 2020. For me, our Good Friday service was particularly special. We had to adapt our normal Good Friday liturgical practices to take account of being 'online'. Instead of including the traditional 'veneration of the Cross' (usual on Good Friday in Roman Catholic and many Anglican churches) we displayed on Zoom a series of images of Jesus, representing different geographical and cultural contexts. The display was very powerful and reflected well the multi-national nature of Holy Trinity's congregation. But interspersed with such displays, and with music and meditations, we could see in a 'Zoom gallery' the faces of our fellow members of Holy Trinity Church – joining the service from their homes in Geneva, France or in some cases much further away. We were, at the time, all wondering what the future was going to hold. The tension was palpably present. I suspect that it was a mercy that none of us, at that moment, really expected the pandemic to continue to blight 'normal' life for as long as it did – and in some ways still does. Alan's lines below catch powerfully that sense of unuttered fear, and the strange mix of community and isolation that worship via Zoom had begun to offer us in April 2020.

From our isolation
we zoom to the Cross,
see one another's faces,
smiles, tears not far away,
joining Christ in his isolation,
finding ourselves reduced to silence
by the exposed anatomy of love.

(Alan Amos)

That Good Friday experience offers a helpful entry point for addressing the question as to how my religious tradition, Christianity, has responded to the Covid pandemic. It illustrates both some of the practical issues and the theological questions posed by my religion and the pandemic to each other.

As its name suggests, the uniqueness of Christianity within the world's religions is largely linked to the place and role it gives to Jesus Christ. Two 'themes' that are both prominent in Christian theology and which the pandemic has interrogated are the incarnation of Christ and the death of Christ. I will look first at the 'incarnation', even though in Christian history it is likely that reflection on the meaning of Jesus's death preceded the development of incarnational theology.

Incarnation: The exposed anatomy of love

The word 'incarnation' is a fundamental term in classical Christian theology. Containing within itself the Latin word *caro* ('flesh') it reflects the key biblical affirmation, 'The word became flesh and dwelt among us' (Jn 1.14). To speak of God 'incarnate' in Jesus Christ is to suggest that in this human being God was uniquely present, that divinity embraced humanity, that eternity entered time, that universality and particularity can complement each other and that what is physical and material can also be holy and a pathway to the spiritual. It is a profoundly paradoxical statement. I would argue that all religion contains an element of paradox, though I think paradox may be particularly significant within Christianity. However, 'the incarnation present[s] us with the supreme paradox' (Baillie 1948: 106). But reflection on the incarnation is not simply reflection on the person of Christ. It has implications for Christ's followers who can be described as 'the body of Christ', and for the nature of Christian worship. A Christian theology of the sacraments – in particular baptism and Holy Communion (or Eucharist) – is ultimately based on the incarnation.

The use of Zoom – as in that Good Friday online worship – forces us to explore a little more deeply what we mean by 'incarnation' and its implications.

It raises new questions about this paradox. For in one sense such digital worship largely removes the physical dimension of 'gathering' together, of being able physically to touch one's fellow worshippers. We are isolated from each other in our separate dwellings which may be geographically far apart. On that Good Friday we could also no longer physically 'touch' that wood of the cross, which was for many an important symbol of the physicality of Christ's death.

And yet in other ways that digital worship was profoundly incarnational and physical. Alan's phrase 'the exposed anatomy of love' caught well the way that our community's mutual sharing of the Zoom screen allowed each of us to be nearer to others than in reality we often were in the church building. We could peer into one another's faces, into each one's hopes and fears. And in that particular Good Friday act of worship the replacement of one physical cross by a range of images of Christ from around the world allowed for another dimension of 'incarnation' to be acknowledged: the fact that incarnation is necessarily linked with particularity, with which contextuality has an intriguing relationship. The human Jesus was a Jewish male who died around 30 CE, but is it 'truer' to the incarnation to depict him solely in these terms, or in ways that 'incarnate' him in the cultures of his modern followers who are far removed from New Testament Palestine in both time and place? Covid did not initiate these questions, but perhaps the digital nature of much worship during this period helped us to continue asking them.

The death of Christ: We Zoom to the cross

The service that Alan's poem was reflecting on was held on Good Friday – the holiest day of the Christian year which commemorates the suffering and death of Jesus Christ, and beginning with its historical reality explores questions about the theological 'meaning[s]' of the event. Classic Christian theology – partly influenced by its Greek philosophical roots – has often sought to distance 'God' from the physical and emotional suffering which was a clear aspect of Christ's passion. Patripassianism, the idea that on the cross God the Father suffers, was regarded as a heresy. The cry from the cross which is on Jesus's lips according to the Gospels of Mark and Matthew, 'My God, my God, why have you forsaken me' (Mt. 27.46; Mk 15.34), has been used to argue that at this moment, as Jesus was, according to classic atonement theologies, paying the price of human sin, God the Father was not participating directly in or responding to his suffering.

There has, however, long been a minority position, linked initially to the name of the twelfth-century Peter Abelard, which has by contrast suggested that God was deeply involved in the suffering both of Christ and of the world. Helen Waddell's classic novel *Peter Abelard* portrays this in story form. Peter and his friend Thibault have found a rabbit caught in a trap, who has been set free but then whimpered and died in Peter's arms:

> Thibault nodded.
> 'I know,' he said. 'Only – I think God is in it too.'
> Abelard looked up sharply.
> 'In it? Do you mean that it makes Him suffer, the way it does us?'
> Again Thibault nodded.
> 'Thibault, do you mean Calvary?'
> Thibault shook his head. 'That was only a piece of it – the piece that we
>   saw – in time. Like that.' He pointed to a fallen tree beside them sawn
>   through the middle.
> 'That dark ring there, it goes up and down the whole length of the tree.
>   But you only see it where it is cut across. That is what Christ's life was;
>   the bit of God that we saw.'
>
> (Waddell [1933] 1947: 264)

The great wars, revolutions and holocausts of the twentieth century meant that the Abelardian understanding that 'God is in it too' have become much more influential in recent years. So in this respect Covid has not actually initiated a major shift in Christian theology. But it has probably accentuated an existing direction of travel. In the face of the widespread suffering over the last two years the sense that God, through the passion of Jesus Christ, could share deeply in human pain was a vital spiritual reassurance for many Christians. All religions find themselves needing to address what is commonly called 'the problem of evil'. The sense that they are treading no darker path than God in Christ has trodden before provides part of a Christian faith-based response to many forms of evil – including the suffering experienced as a result of Covid. One of the features of our Covid times has, as Alan's poem suggests, been the isolation experienced by many. With this Jesus's own sense of forsakenness on the cross deeply resonated.

An intriguing development however, in part linked to the above, is that the pandemic has led to a renewed interest among some Christians in the language and theology of lament. By 'lament' I mean a sharp, impassioned form of protest to God against perceived injustice and a demand that God address this situation.

Although 'laments' appear quite widely within the Hebrew Bible including prophetic literature, Job and the book of Psalms, and Jesus's own words on the Cross from Ps. 22.1 are an expression of lament – Christian spirituality has, certainly in mainstream Western churches, been hesitant about 'lament'. It is not considered polite to speak to God in this way! The pandemic has, however, produced a considerable amount of interest in biblical laments and their implications for us in these times, including a resurgence of interest in the book of Job.

Communion and sacrament: 'From our isolation'

Good Friday is actually the one day in the year when it is traditional in many churches not to celebrate Holy Communion. The day is concentrated on Christ's passion itself – rather than on Holy Communion, which is, inter alia, a memorial of that passion. But for the part of the Christian spectrum with which I am most associated, broadly liturgical in style and in which the Holy Communion is normally now the central act of worship, Covid, especially in the early period of 'total lockdown' was a real challenge – although one which eventually resulted in considerable creative reflection. For Holy Communion by its very sacramental nature involves the consecration and sharing of physical elements such as bread and wine, which could contain additional health risks even in situations where it was possible to hold in-person worship.

Early in the pandemic period Michael Curry, Presiding Bishop of The Episcopal Church (TEC), wrote to members of his Church 'On Our Theology of Worship' in response to the problems posed (Office of Public Affairs 2020). His letter was critical of some of the solutions offered, such as 'drive-thru' Eucharists. He also drew attention to the fact that until fairly recently the most widely used form of Anglican public worship was the Daily Office, Morning and Evening Prayer, rather than Holy Communion and suggested that '[u]nder our present circumstances, in making greater use of the Office there may be an opportunity to recover aspects of our tradition that point to the sacramentality of the scriptures, the efficacy of prayer itself, the holiness of the household as the "domestic church"'.

In Holy Trinity Geneva, the worshipping community with which I was most associated in the early period of the pandemic, online Sunday worship did indeed begin by using Morning Prayer, but fairly quickly, as we realized that worshipping online was not going to be merely short term, the question of how to hold online services of Holy Communion was raised. Although there was a certain amount of nervousness about what was happening among the central Church of England hierarchy, permission was granted for priests to preside at 'Holy Communion' in their own homes, where possible with a member of their family present. As practised in my own experience, those physically present with the priest received the consecrated bread and wine: those participating via Zoom were invited to make a 'spiritual communion' in the form of a prayer. Initially the prayer used for this purpose was a traditional Roman Catholic one by St Alphonse Liguori, but its rather baroque language did not sit easily with our Anglican ethos, and my husband Alan wrote an alternative version which spoke of 'being present together in heart and mind at this holy communion … ; as we unite with one another from the places where we are, may your communion be fulfilled in us now through the work of the life-giving Holy Spirit' (Amos 2021). This prayer has been adopted by several other Anglican church communities and continues to be used.

The exigencies of the pandemic however provoked further (and ongoing) discussion about the nature of Holy Communion. Richard Burridge, a well-known British New Testament scholar, drew an online circle around himself, in which eventually the question was raised, 'I have been wondering who to ask … what is the range of consecration?' In other words, could the words of consecration said by a priest sitting in front of one Zoom screen, be efficacious in consecrating bread and wine held up by a lay participant sitting in front of another Zoom screen? Drawing on his experience of online services, Burridge has recently published a book in which this question is aired (Burridge 2022a, 2022b).

In this last section of my reflection the word 'communion' (and associated words) has appeared several times, and with several different resonances. 'Communion' (*koinonia* in Greek) is a key word in Christian vocabulary. Its overlapping and ambiguous range of meanings is both a theological resource and a challenge. The pandemic has challenged us to explore what 'communion' may mean: in our worship with our church community in person and online, in our 'communion' with fellow human beings in far off lands given issues such as the inequity of global vaccine distribution, in the responses made by some of our national leadership, both religious and political, which have at times felt inadequate and deeply lacking in 'communion'.

One last – and rather different – point. I asked a friend, of a different theological tradition to my own, what she thought the pandemic had taught Christians. She thought that it spoke to her of the responsiveness yet unexpectedness of God. As she put it, 'Christians have been praying to God in relation to the ecological crisis. The pandemic could be viewed as part of God's answer to this prayer. It has been a time when the use of fossil fuels have considerably decreased, and when people have had time to reflect how their ways of living have been harming our planet, and perhaps – just perhaps – resolve to do things differently in the future.' Amen to that.

References

Amos, Clare (2021). 'Bread of Life'. 21 July. Accessible online at URL: https://faithineurope.net/page/4.

Baillie, Donald M. (1948). *God Was in Christ*. New York: Charles Scribner's Sons.

Burridge, Richard A. (2022a). *Holy Communion in Contagious Times*. Eugene, OR: Cascade Books.

Burridge, Richard A. (2022b). 'Is a Zoom Rite a Valid Form of Communion?'. *Church Times*. 21 January. Accessible online at URL: https://www.churchtimes.co.uk/articles/2022/21-january/comment/opinion/is-a-zoom-rite-a-valid-form-of-communion.

Office of Public Affairs (2020). 'Presiding Bishop Michael Curry's Word to the Church: On Our Theology of Worship'. 31 March. Accessible online at URL: www.episcopalchurch.org/publicaffairs/presiding-bishop-michael-currys-word-to-the-church-on-our-theology-of-worship.

Waddell, Helen ([1933] 1947). *Peter Abelard*. London: Henry Holt.

5

We can't forget: Conservative Protestants in the Covid-19 pandemic

Camille Kaminski Lewis

Since March 2020, the United States has lost a million people to the Covid virus. This tiny airborne pathogen has already killed more Americans than all our country's wars ('How America', 2022). And like all our neighbours, my own faith community of conservative evangelical Protestants in the United States seems to have already forgotten the virus, consumed with the busyness of 'worship' and the comfort of 'getting back to normal'. Evangelicals make up the largest share of American Christians at 25 per cent (Pew Research Center 2014), and so our reaction is largely an American reaction. We are, after all, a loud and united part of the larger whole.

When this pandemic started and I had stockpiled my share of dried beans, pasta and canned tuna for the months ahead, I resorted to my usual coping mechanism in a crisis: historical research. After all, maybe my grandparents and their neighbours from the 1918 pandemic learned a few things that could help us persist. I picked up Alfred E. Crosby's history, and the title should have clued me in ahead of time: *America's Forgotten Pandemic*. Americans a century earlier did terrible job of remembering the H1N1 'Spanish' flu. Crosby called it a lack of 'awe' and 'fear' that let us forget. Our popular press actually documented more about baseball in those years than it did about that deadly virus. And in school, we Americans still study more about Europe's Black Plague from the fourteenth century than about our own in the twentieth. At the time the *New York Times* surmised that because the majority of the flu victims were the same age as the victims of the First World War, we folded the military conflict into the biological one ('Topics' 1918; Crosby 2003: 320–3). But now in the twenty-first century, before the pandemic is even endemic, we are already forgetting, and I think that my faith community of conservative Protestants gives us a clue as to exactly how Americans so easily forget.

Early in the pandemic – before vaccines were available even in drug trials – my evangelical pastor friends amplified one particular Calvinistic Baptist seminarian. Costi Hinn wrote 'Navigating Different COVID-19 Recovery Convictions', for the Midwestern Seminary concluding that 'grace' is what's needed in to combat a viral threat. 'Grace', or courteous forgetting, will help us fight a biological threat. He purrs in the end, 'choose love'. How charming! Who wouldn't want some love in the middle of a worldwide crisis?

But look closer at his text:

> I believe one of the ways that the enemy will seek to divide our ranks within the church is by tempting us to use our opinions against each other. If the Devil has his way, we'll be throwing stones of accusation from all sides, calling the cautious people 'soft,' labeling the optimists of being 'reckless.' More than that, the enemy especially loves when we cement ourselves in political corners; adding opinionated fuel to the already tumultuous fire of conflict.

He continues:

> As the spiral of opinion leads you downward, you must formulate a game plan that takes you upward. It's okay to be different! To have a healthy family, a healthy team, and a healthy church there must [be] room for different opinions and experiences. These differences often stretch us and help us grow together and learn from each other. We need to respect one another and realize that *everyone* [emphasis in original] is navigating a new frontier.

He is talking with 'leadership teams' here which, among evangelicals (particularly those who insist that baptism must be by immersion and only for believers who can personally affirm their faith), is consistently an all-white male pastoral staff. These good guys get thwarted by the devil and those with 'opinions' which 'dominate' and 'spiral downward'. Good guys vs. the Devil, ministers with grace vs. people with opinions, looking up vs. spinning down – this old Southern duel persists in conservative evangelical narratives, and this one is no different (C. Lewis 2021: 40–4).

To his fellow ministers, this preacher asks his public to 'agree to disagree' on science and rise above those troublemakers who will only 'divide our ranks'. Different conclusions in the midst of a pandemic are merely 'convictions' – fundamentalist code for pietistic preferences. Do you drink alcohol socially or abstain? Do you worship with a drum set or a pipe organ? Do you watch PG-13 movies or only G-rated family films? These are the kinds of endless conflicts that Hinn groups together with the public health realities in a pandemic. Do you see wearing a mask as 'soft', or do you see refusing a mask as 'reckless'? Do you participate in congregational singing, or do you believe these 'super spreader' events must wait for a later date? These clashes are all the same kinds of 'convictions', and Hinn and his grace-filled white male team stand outside the debate entirely. They won't get involved. Their indifference to the nitty-gritty is, Hinn claims, 'choosing love'.

They have no skin in the game. Their hands are clean. Their lungs, they presume, are virus-free. Hinn and his team are 'godly' which, in practice, means body-less. It takes forgetting our own humanity to get to that point. We have to forget we have bodies because bodies are vulnerable, messy and (unfortunately) human! And 'only by forgetting', as Nietzsche concludes, can we 'live with any repose, security, and consistency' (Nietzsche 1979: 86). Forgetting brings a kind of 'peace', and, as Nietzsche eventually argues, allows the Übermensch to 'lead'. Hinn admits that he just wants to preserve relationships since 'people matter over opinion'. But the 'people' that matter are not scientists, not public health officials, not the elderly, not women, not the immune-compromised, and not children. Hinn does not even mention Jesus.

A few months after Hinn's relegation of public health rules as mere 'convictions', another white Calvinistic Baptist minister was even more defiant. California fundamentalist and Bob-Jones-University-bred John MacArthur does, at least, start with Jesus. But notice the action he ascribes to his presumed Saviour:

> Christ is Lord of all. He is the one true head of the church. He is also King of kings – sovereign over every earthly authority. Grace Community Church has always stood immovably on those biblical principles. As His people, we are subject to His will and commands as revealed in Scripture. Therefore, we cannot and will not acquiesce to a government-imposed moratorium on our weekly congregational worship or other regular corporate gatherings. Compliance would be disobedience to our Lord's clear commands.
>
> (MacArthur 2020)

MacArthur does not make Jesus an actor. Jesus is not doing anything. He simply is – like a totem. And by the third paragraph, Jesus is nothing more than an object of the preposition [emphasis mine]:

> A father's authority is limited to his own family. Church leaders' authority (which is delegated to them *by Christ*) is limited to church matters. And government is specifically tasked with the oversight and protection of civic peace and well-being within the boundaries of a nation or community.

The whole narrative is centred around the white male authority in the family and the church which has been ordained *by Christ* which acts against the government. MacArthur, like Hinn, ignores the vulnerable, the old (other 80-somethings like himself) and the educated.

Consistently in these evangelical narratives, the white male church leaders are the heroes of their own story, the solitary actors, an American evangelical version of Nietzsche's Übermensch. All the others with their convictions are either ugly adversaries or mere scenery, wallpaper on the set of the white ministerial drama, seconds in the duel between preachers and the devil of government (C. Lewis 2021: 40–4).

It has been a brutal two years for all of us. And in American evangelical churches, when we needed each other the most, when we had a perfect opportunity to demonstrate neighbourly care, or as my pastor says, to 'be incarnational', too many evangelical leaders like Hinn and MacArthur raged that carrying on as usual was the only godly thing (A. Lewis). In order to carry on as usual – to continue meeting in person, to ignore mask-mandates and social distancing – they had to forget that we are all equally frail, untidy bodies who need care.

Covid-19 has highlighted existing social inequalities. Communities of Black and Brown folks have been hit the hardest. Material differences are made more different. And in the process, the immaterial differences are even more stark. If you worship in a community that amplifies the words of Hinn and MacArthur, obeying mask mandates puts you in the enemy's camp, and getting a vaccine – as was irrationally yelled at me around my KN95 mask in my own church lobby – makes you a cruel, anti-life pagan. And it is not just the lay person on Sunday morning who gets heat. When renowned Southern Baptist leader Russell Moore along with Walter Kim, President of the National Association of Evangelicals, confronted the evangelical penchant to believe the wildest conspiracy theories about the Covid vaccine, only a few months passed before Moore left the employ of that evangelical denomination.

Forgetting all these bruhahas would be the easiest, but it's not the best. We do want to forget the brutality of a million deaths, of Zoomed holidays, of toilet paper and baby formula shortages, of hours-long waits for Covid testing. And we also want to forget this polarization between Red America and Blue, between science-affirmers and self-affirmers, between those of us who have bodies and those of us who don't want to admit that we do. In forgetting, there is the veneer of peace with the white male leaders repeating the story of their own heroic deeds against their enemy, the government.

As I was growing up, my father regularly told the story of his older brother's death in the 1918 pandemic. Because my grandmother had escaped an abusive arranged marriage in Poland by riding steerage to the United States, she had not yet married my grandfather when their first son was born. And because of that, she had not yet baptized my uncle in the Catholic Church. And because of all that, my grandparents' priest told her that my uncle was in Hell. That white-male-centric declaration changed everything for her. She left Catholicism and became a Russellite because the Russellites told her she would see her son again in the Resurrection. ('Russellites' was the name given to Charles Taze Russell's Bible Students, now better known as Jehovah's Witnesses.) They saw her pain and suffering and the brutality of her situation and gave her hope. My father telling that story his whole life and my whole life changed me. His remembering changed me. I learned in that story that leader-centred religion is abusive and the opposite of faith. I learned that God knows we have bodies that are frail and virus-prone. I learned to persist through false, leader-centric pontifications. I learned that we all need hope.

My faith community of conservative Protestants, like all of America in 2022 and in 1918, has attempted to make sense of the pandemic by forgetting, because in that forgetting, we presume, we can have peace. But it is a disruptive, unhealthy, shallow and hopeless peace.

Covid was a Lenten fast, an observance that remembers that Jesus himself had a body which needed food and water. We cannot forget our fast. We have to remember the nitty-gritty daily existence of double-masking, of fogged-up glasses, of sharing at-home Covid tests with our friends who forgot to order their share. We have to remember sanitation theatre, repeated 'you're on mute' pleas, and the longing for a hug or a handshake. We have to remember the sourdough recipes, the Netflix viewing parties, the sea-shanty songs, the virtual choirs and the at-home sewing marathons so we could donate fabric masks to shelters, schools and nursing homes. If we forget, we are conceding authority to the gnostic-ish, body-ignoring, science-denying, übermensch-like religious leaders. If we remember, we can underline God's care, our persistence and best practices for our future. In remembering we can have hope.

References

Crosby, A. (2003). *America's Forgotten Pandemic: The Influenza of 1918*. New York: Cambridge University Press.

Hinn, C. (2020). 'Navigating Different COVID-19 Recovery Convictions'. *For the Church*. 27 April 2020. Accessible online at URL: https://ftc.co/resource-library/blog-entries/navigating-different-covid-19-recovery-convictions/.

'How America Reached One Million COVID Deaths'. (2022). *New York Times*. 13 May 2022. Accessible online at URL: https://www.nytimes.com/interactive/2022/05/13/us/covid-deaths-us-one-million.html.

Lewis, A. (2020). 'Philosophy of Ministry'. *Mitchell Road Presbyterian Church*. Accessible online at URL: https://www.mitchellroad.org/philosophy.

Lewis, C. (2021). '"The Bounds of Their Habitation": Bob Jones' Rhetorical Duel with Billy Graham'. *Fides et Historia*, 53 (1) 37–59.

MacArthur, J. (2020). 'Christ, Not Caesar Is the Head of the Church'. *Grace Church*. 24 July 2020. Accessible online at URL: https://www.gracechurch.org/news/posts/1988.

Moore, R. and Kim, W. (2021). 'Not the Mark of the Beast: Evangelicals Should Fight Conspiracy Theories and Welcome the Vaccines'. *Washington Post*, 24 February 2021. Accessible online at URL: https://www.washingtonpost.com/religion/2021/02/24/evangelicals-covid-vaccine-russell-moore-walter-kim/.

Nietzsche, F. W. and Breazeale, D. (1979). *Philosophy and Truth: Selections from Nietzsche's Notebooks of the Early 1870's*. Atlantic Highlands, NJ: Humanities Press.

Pew Research Center (2014). 'Religious Landscape Study'. Accessible online at URL https://www.pewresearch.org/religion/religious-landscape-study/.

'Topics of the Times' (5 November 1918). *New York Times*, 12.

6

'What people's hands have earned': Islamic perspectives on Covid

Usama Hasan

Why do pandemics happen?

A common Muslim saying is that *the world is a place of test*. Whether good or bad things happen to us, they are a test from God: in *good* times, to see if we will be *grateful*; in *bad* times, to see if we will be *patient*. This is a repeated Qur'anic theme, for example:

> We test you with evil and goodness, as a trial!
>
> (*The Prophets*, 21:35)

> Do they not see that they are tested every year, once or twice: yet they neither repent nor reflect?
>
> (*Repentance*, 9:126)

Furthermore, trials and tribulations befall humanity partly as a result of our own misdeeds. As brutal as this may sound, it is an aspect of Reality (itself, a name of God in Islamic tradition) in which Muslims have firm faith. This again is a key Qur'anic theme:

> Corruption has become manifest, in land and on sea, because of what people's hands have earned, that He (God) may make them taste some of what they have done, that they may return.
>
> (*The Romans*, 30:41)

Were God to take people to account for what they have earned, He would not leave a single creature on the face of the earth, but He grants them respite until a term appointed.

(*Originator*, 35:45)

Beware a trial that will not specifically afflict the wrongdoers amongst you, and know that God is severe in retribution.

(*Spoils of War*, 8:25)

At the time of writing, scientists are still divided over whether the Covid-19 global pandemic was caused by a 'lab leak' or by human consumption of mammals kept in unhygienic conditions. Either way, many Muslims have regarded the pandemic as a test, punishment and admonition from God towards humanity: a reminder that a microscopic microbe can cause such devastation to human life and wealth. These momentous events have happened 'that God may know those who have faith, and select martyrs from amongst you' (*The Family of Amram*, 3:140), for those who die of plague and other unexpected calamities are regarded as martyrs in Islam.

Revival of Islamic teachings about dealing with plagues

Canonical Islamic sources of Hadith record that the Prophet Muhammad taught: If you hear of plague in a land, do not travel there. If it occurs in your land, do not leave, fleeing from it.

This is extraordinary advice from the seventh century CE, and one which was revived to good effect by Muslim organizations, authorities and states worldwide, providing religious legitimacy to social distancing and lockdown rules during the pandemic.

An even more subtle insight is gained from a related story from the same era: Caliph Omar was travelling in an expedition to Syria from Medina. On the way, news reached them of the plague of Emmaus in Syria. He consulted his advisors, and one of them testified that he had heard the above teaching from the Prophet, so Omar announced that they would immediately return to Medina. Abu Ubaydah bin al-Jarrah, one of the Caliph's senior advisors, questioned him, apparently because he had not heard this teaching directly himself and was not convinced of its authenticity:

'Are we fleeing from the decree of God?'

Abu Ubaydah's fatalism was so strong that he apparently favoured completing the journey and submitting to the will of God, even if that meant disease or death. But Caliph Omar replied brilliantly:

'We are fleeing from the decree of God to the decree of God.'

In other words, Caliph Omar understood deeply that everything is the decree of God – this is a rather obvious consequence of a monotheistic belief in One, Omniscient God who knows the past, present and future. This Islamic certainty has guided many Muslims through the immense tribulation of the Covid pandemic.

The pandemic's impact on Islamic religious practice

A central Islamic practice is that of the five daily prayers, with prayer services held at every local mosque. The Covid lockdowns affected these enormously: mosques closed their doors to their regular congregations, although many continued to hold small prayer services in order to symbolically keep the mosques open and functioning throughout the pandemic.

The first lockdowns around the world, including in the UK, were brought in around a month before Ramadan, the month of fasting. Ramadan is a month-long festival of fasting, eating and worship. Large crowds gather daily to eat together at the beginning and end of the daily fast, and to offer extra prayers together in mosques. Attendance at the five-times-daily and Friday prayers rockets throughout Ramadan. There is also a special practice of spiritual seclusion or retreat in mosques, when millions of men, and occasionally women, remain confined to the mosque in close company with others during its last ten days.

This carried many public health risks during the Covid pandemic, especially in developing countries where many poor people rely on the Ramadan charitable practice of feeding people to eat two meals per day. Governments of countries with large Muslim populations faced a crisis of decision-making and social acceptance around Covid policy. In Ramadan, extra prayer services are held in mosques that also host daily communal breaking of the fast in the evenings. The threatened disruption to Ramadan activities led leading Islamic clerics in Pakistan to defy the government lockdown and announce that daily, nightly and Friday prayers would resume for Ramadan. This led to negotiations with the government, resulting in a 20-point plan agreed with the dissenting clerics for a managed opening of Pakistan's mosques in time for Ramadan and

Eid, the festival of the breaking of the fast. The mosques would continue their activities, but with social distancing, masks, increased cleaning and other precautions in place. The theologians argued successfully that shopping malls remained open and were thronged with customers: it would be utterly wrong to close places of worship whilst markets flourished, especially during the holy month.

In addition to the daily cycle of prayers, we have the large congregational prayers on Friday afternoons. In countries with strict lockdowns, many preachers switched to giving Friday sermons online, thus opening up access to new congregants who were otherwise unable to attend mosque physically. The latter included people with disabilities, mothers and even women in general, since unfortunately many mosques do not have equal facilities for them. This development has left a lasting legacy in terms of increasing inclusion at mosque, going forward.

Mosques often rely on their daily and weekly congregations for funding through donations, especially in countries without state control or supervision of religion. Thus, the lockdowns were financially damaging although increased online activities and donations may have compensated somewhat for this.

Another important prayer service is that of funeral prayers. This service is performed at mosque or cemetery, followed by burial. For those unable to join the funeral service, there is a disputed practice of offering funeral prayers *in absentia* of the deceased: people can offer funeral prayers at another mosque or at home, praying for the soul of the dearly departed even though they are very distant from the funeral itself. Necessity being the mother of invention, this latter practice has increased in popularity during the Covid era, and many Muslim funerals have been live-streamed for the first time.

The annual Hajj pilgrimage to Mecca

Within two months of the end of Ramadan, Saudi Arabia hosts the Hajj, or annual pilgrimage to Mecca, an essential pillar of Islamic practice. Every healthy Muslim who can afford it is expected to perform the Hajj at least once in their lifetime. Ramadan and Hajj are related: the two Eid festivals are associated with these two periods of worship, and Ramadan is seen as preparation for those intending to embark on the Hajj.

The Hajj is usually attended by about two and a half million people, almost two million of whom are foreign visitors. Pilgrims come from every country in the world, and the Saudis solve a large and complex logistical problem every year in accommodating them. For countries with large Muslim populations, the Saudis impose a quota of one pilgrim per 1,000 Muslims in that country.

For an entire week, huge crowds crisscross Mecca and its surrounding plains daily in observance of complicated Hajj rituals. Most of them also spend a week or two in Medina, the city of the Prophet. During the pandemic, it was very difficult to see how this could be kept up safely: Mecca and Medina were already under strict lockdown and curfew.

To give a sense of the enormity of this decision affecting the journey of millions to their spiritual home and holiest sanctuary, the Hajj has been cancelled or become very difficult to attend many times in Islamic history due to war, natural disasters and plagues. But it has never, during the century-long Saudi rule over Mecca, been cancelled. Although there was speculation in Western media that the Hajj might be cancelled in 2020, the Saudis were reluctant to cancel the Hajj completely, just as they had exempted the Holy Mosques of Mecca and Medina from the nationwide closure of mosques due to Covid-19: small prayer services were still being held daily at the two Holy Mosques, with scanners installed to monitor people's body temperatures as part of the fight against coronavirus.

The Saudis have reduced pilgrim numbers before: the number in 2013 was almost 40 per cent down on the previous year due to restrictions imposed because of a large-scale construction project at the Sacred Mosque in Mecca. Given the above considerations and constraints, the Hajj did go ahead in 2020, but with a vastly reduced number of pilgrims, stripped back to allow no foreigners: only a thousand Saudis who had tested negative for the coronavirus, including royalty and senior clerics, were able to perform the Hajj. In 2021, the number of pilgrims was increased to sixty thousand, and the Hajj was only open to Saudi nationals and residents. In 2022, the number was further increased to a million pilgrims, including foreign visitors, but still less than half the pre-pandemic numbers.

Striking a balance between religious practice and pandemic precautions

The dilemma that Saudi authorities faced is one which many Islamic leaders have grappled with: how to strike a balance between fulfilling their obligations to their faith and their communities while acting responsibly in the battle to contain the spread of the coronavirus, a battle in which religious authorities can play a vital, and maybe even a decisive, role.

Indeed, imams around the world have urged Muslim communities to obey government and health agencies, as preservation of life is an essential Islamic principle. They have also helped to counter religion-based misinformation and misleading advice regarding the pandemic. Such fake news has included mutually contradictory claims that the pandemic was simultaneously God's punishment for non-believers as well as a non-Muslim conspiracy against Islam due to the closure of mosques and severe restrictions on the Hajj. The misinformation also extended to discouraging vaccination, despite the centuries-strong Islamic tradition of developing medicine and hospitals.

It is important for political leaders and health agencies to work with religious leaders on such matters. A case in point is the otherwise excellent World Health Organization (WHO) guidance on Ramadan in 2020, at the height of the pandemic, that included a problematic line asking authorities to 'provide alcohol-based hand-rub (at least 70 per cent alcohol) at the entrance to and inside mosques'. Given that hundreds of millions of Muslims believe that alcohol is ritually impure and prohibited to drink or even handle, this had the potential to undermine the guidance and even cause social unrest, because there were loud and influential voices who would accuse authorities of promoting physical impurity and uncleanliness inside mosques.

To mitigate this concern, the WHO should have referred to the many religious and fatwa-issuing authorities who had endorsed the use of alcohol-based hand-rubs in the Covid-19 situation as a case of dire necessity due to the Qur'anic principle that necessity allows even what is usually prohibited. This would have been a good example of governments, health agencies and religious leaders working together against a lethal threat to everyone.

In multifaith societies, interfaith dialogue and cooperation is the essence of human existence whether it is on a local level with cooperation to assist needy neighbours or on a national scale, such as governments working with leaders of many religions to promote public health messages via faith communities. Over the past two years since the Covid-19 pandemic began, I have seen the beauty of interfaith cooperation where I live as Muslims, Christians and people of other faiths or no faith in my local area have worked together to run food banks and baby banks for those less fortunate.

Islamic marriages

Islamic marriage ceremonies, which are often performed at mosques but can be done at home or other suitable venue, have also been affected by the pandemic. Due to lockdowns, many marriage parties were very small and limited to people's homes and gardens. As an imam, I officiate in dozens of such ceremonies every year. I met a grandfather at one of these small wedding parties who was encouraging his grandchildren to get married during lockdown, since they would save a fortune by having small wedding parties!

I also officiated in some marriage ceremonies with the bare minimum audience allowed by the UK government's 'rule of six': the bride and groom, and their parents. (As someone providing professional services, I was classified as a worker, not a member of the wedding party, so was able to be the seventh person present.) Couples getting married have also used technology to allow family and friends to participate in their lockdown wedding parties via video-conference. I have also actually conducted several dozen Islamic weddings via video call around the world since the pandemic began.

Conclusion

Islamic practice has been irreversibly transformed by the rapid adoption of technology forced by the necessity of the Covid pandemic. A welcome effect of this is the inclusion and participation of non-traditional worshippers and congregants. The pandemic has also increased our sense of mortality, especially as we mourn our Covid martyrs, and the importance of treasuring what is most important to us: family, friends, community and the most sacred value of all: our relationship with God.

References

References are from The Holy Qur'an, and are the author's own translation.

7

Glimpses into Islamic perspectives and practice

Farhana Mayer

Worship

The daily rites of Islam involve canonical prayers to be performed at dawn (*ṣalāt al-fajr*), midday (*ṣalāt al-ẓuhr*), mid-afternoon (*ṣalāt al-ʿaṣr*), evening (*ṣalāt al-maghrib*) and at night *(salat al-ʿishāʾ)*. Many Muslims consider it meritorious to perform these five daily prayers in congregation at a mosque; men are expected to attend the Friday midday mosque prayer and sermon. However, the canonical prayers may all be performed at home, or anywhere convenient when on the move. A Muslim does not need a cleric, a mosque or a fully functioning society, to be able to fulfil his or her religious rites; any adequately healthy person can perform the required worship wherever possible. One needs God's presence, one's own presence of mind (much harder to find and maintain), and some quiet space. Muslims also perform supererogatory acts of worship, including Qur'an-recitation and invocations of the Divine names (*asmāʾ Allāh al-Ḥusnā*). This worship too requires only God, scripture, self and some quiet space. In short, Islamic worship is suited to both individual and congregational performance. From this point of view, the shift – for compliance with Covid restrictions – to all prayers being done at home was not difficult. The local Friday sermon by Imam Monawar Hussain (Muslim Chaplain, Oxford University Hospitals, NHS Foundation Trust) was delivered online or by radio. But mosque attendance is not just about prayers; it has the value of exchange of community news in person, and suchlike; this was lost.

Ramadan, the holy month of fasting, can also be a sociable time normally, with people coming together to break the fast and gathering in mosques for extra night-time prayers. Nonetheless, Ramadan too can be observed at home. According to Imam Monawar, one positive impact of the pandemic and lockdowns was that for two consecutive Ramadans, Muslim men who normally go to the mosque for the extra Ramadan night prayers while their womenfolk stay at home, were praying at home with their families. This, then, was one way in which a shift from congregational worship to home worship enhanced family religious life during Covid. Something I personally experienced in isolation and lockdowns was the easy expansion – based on passages such as Qur'an surah 73 and Islamic spiritual practices like supererogatory prayers (nawāfil) and invocations of God's Names (dhikr) – of the regular Islamic rituals into practically a monastic schedule of prayers, intercessory invocations and meditations.

Theological considerations: Who is responsible for the pandemic, God or humankind?

People have asked me why God allowed the pandemic to happen, tracing this crisis back to God, the All-Powerful. However, a spectrum of Muslims immediately looked to humankind's actions as the cause. Both stances are grounded in scripture. From the first chapter, the Qur'an inculcates a keen sense of human accountability, and readers are frequently reminded throughout the Book of being answerable to God Himself. There are also over sixty-one Qur'anic verses which speak of the deeds and outcomes which people 'have earned' by their actions ('deeds done' are often described in the Qur'an as what people's 'hands have earned' or have 'already presented'). Among the verses which place the responsibility for difficulties that afflict people on humankind is Q. 30:41 (in the chapter entitled al-Rūm, 'Byzantium'), which states, 'corruption has appeared on land and in the sea because of what the hands of people have earned, so that He makes them taste/experience some of what they have done in order that they might turn back [from doing bad]'. Similarly, Q. 42:30 (al-Shūrā, 'Consultation') states, 'Whatever difficulty afflicts you it is because of what your hands have earned; yet He (God) forgives much.' Applying this to Covid, though the virus may have been a natural phenomenon, its transfer to people and hence the pandemic seem likely to have been the result of human activity (Felter 2021; Lowe 2022); the logical and scriptural follow-on being that people should change the practices that led to the pandemic. On the other hand, Q. 4:78 (al-Nisā', 'Women') states categorically that good and bad are both from God: 'When some good befalls them, they say, "This is from God" but when something bad befalls them, they say, "This is from you (Muḥammad)". Say, "All is from God".' This can be interpreted to mean that the pandemic is an 'act of God'. Setting aside questions to do with Divine Command Theory (see Malik 2021), the following theological questions arise: If it is God who sends good and ill to creatures, can people freely choose between doing good or evil? If not, how can they be accountable for their doings? If people do freely choose their actions and are responsible for them, does that mean people create their deeds? If so, does this impact God's status as sole creator? And since God is almighty and good and can, if He chooses, intervene at will in earthly matters, why does evil happen on earth, especially things that may seem to be 'acts of God', like the Covid pandemic?

Regarding the first four questions, the key points that Sunni Muslim scholastic discussions have historically debated are whether God's omnipotence and singularity-as-Creator are compromised by the needs for justice and regard for human free will and responsibility (Watt 2012; Campanini 2012). The Mu'tazilite theologians notably pointed out that if humanity is to be punished for things they did not produce, then that would be unjust, whereas Q. 45:22 (al-Jāthiyah, 'Kneeling') states 'God created the heavens and the earth in truth with justice (bi'l-Ḥaqq) so that each soul be requited for what it earned/acquired/gained (kasabat), and they shall not be treated unjustly'. Therefore, as famously declared by the Mu'tazilites many centuries ago, humankind must have free will and be responsible for their deeds (Campanini 2012). The Ash'arite theologians provided an interesting resolution to the dilemma. Based on the verb kasaba which means 'to earn; acquire; gain', their concept of iktisāb ('acquisition') entailed that people 'acquire' deeds (Bearman et al 2012). In other words, while all deeds are created by God, people acquire the merit of doing good or the demerit of doing evil by choosing which deeds to perform. This accommodates human choice while safeguarding God's singular status as Creator and recognizing that He is not the perpetrator of evil. A distinction between human perpetration of evil and divine act is also found in Q. 29:10 (al-'Ankabūt, 'The Spider') which cautions against equating trials emanating from people with punishment from God.

The last question (on God's intervention) underscores the weight of human responsibility. The Islamic concept of humankind as the stewards or successors placed by God on earth (khalīfah/khalā'if fi'l-arḍ) – for example in Q. 2:30–4 (al-Baqarah, 'The Cow') and in Q. 6:165 (al-An'ām, 'Livestock') – comes with commensurate responsibility. Every person is responsible for his or her deeds and the consequences of what their hands have acquired; see, for example, Q. 6:164 (al-An'ām, 'Livestock') and Q. 14:51 (Ibrāhīm, 'Abraham'). Direct divine intervention on earth obviously is not the norm. Rather, heavenly help comes through revelatory guidance and in strengthening goodness in people, God thus working on earth through humankind. For Muslims, the 'Most Beautiful Names of God' (Q. 7:180, al-A'rāf, 'The Mountain Heights';

17:110, al-Isrāʾ, 'The Night Journey'; 20:8, Ṭāʾ Hāʾ; 59:22–24, al-Ḥashr, 'The Gathering'), which regularly punctuate the Qur'an, enshrine attributes of God and ethical principles, many of which humanity could seek to emulate (Burrell and Daher 1995). The idea of evoking God's attributes through invoking His names and choosing to live in alignment with the principles they present has the existential impact of empowering people to live and function in an ethically sound way. In this qualitative manner, God regularly 'intervenes'. Nonetheless, Muslims believe He does work miracles too. But the when, how and why of His interventions are His merciful and wise decisions.

Challenges of Covid: Suffering loss, hurt and death

Several Qur'anic verses reveal the religious instincts of accepting that death is a certainty and that life on earth is itself a testing time and will present the trials of pain, sorrow, affliction, injury, loss and bereavement. This is stated categorically in Q. 2:153–7 (al-Baqarah, 'The Cow'), wherein people of faith are also encouraged to resort to prayer and patience in testing times:

> O those who believe! Seek help in patient perseverance and prayer; verily, God is with the patient/steadfast. And do not call those who are killed in God's way 'dead'; nay, (they are) living but you do not perceive it. And We shall test you with something of fear and hunger and loss of property, life and gains; but give glad tidings to the patient/steadfast, those who, when a calamity befalls them, say, 'We belong to God and indeed to Him we are returning'. [157]Upon those (people) are blessings and mercy from your Lord; those people, they are the rightly-guided.
>
> (Q. 2:153–157.)

Several other scriptural passages speak of trials through both good things and difficult things (Q. 21:35, al-Anbiyāʾ, 'the Prophets'), and of the trials of death and life being part of life to ascertain 'which of you is best in deeds' (67:2, al-Mulk, Sovereignty). Q. 2:214 (al-Baqarah, 'The Cow') asks if people think they will enter Paradise without being touched by hardship and affliction like those before them were. Together with this come the reassurances that God is 'the Mighty, the Forgiving' (67:2) and that 'God's help is near' (2:214). Moreover, some verses imply that people should not expect full requital for their efforts during their time on earth; 'you will receive in full your recompense on the day of resurrection' (Q. 3:185, āl ʿImrān, 'The People of ʿImrān'). Without denying the hardship of trials, such teachings infuse a degree of resilience in believers, providing comfort and strength in times of loss, injury and grief. Furthermore, Muslims are expected to do their bit in tackling trials, alleviating difficulties, and, in appropriate ways, righting wrongs – a Prophetic narration states that if a Muslim witnesses something that is not right he or she should seek to rectify it either in action or word or thought (*An-Nawawi*' 1997: Hadith #34). Imams and Muslim doctors made a point of disseminating reliable information on Covid vaccines for those who had questions. Supplementing state support, Muslims, like other faith communities, provided, as best they could in the circumstances, appropriate support for those in isolation, ill with Covid, bereaved, affected by the economic repercussions of the pandemic and, not least, for burying the dead.

Dealing with death

There are many Islamic rituals and social conventions around death and burial, which provide the bereaved with tremendous support and help them achieve closure. Extended family and community gather daily to pray and recite the Qur'an together for the first week and again on the fortieth day. Family and friends cater for the bereaved family, allowing the latter space to simply mourn. Mosque staff and trained volunteers take the lead in the obligatory ritual ablution (*ghusl*) of the body prior to burial; the bereaved may participate in this if they choose, and the guidance of those trained in this service is indispensable for the bereaved family. All this was stripped away by Covid and lockdowns. This deprivation means healing closure will take longer to achieve.

In hospital

During lockdown much of the religious provision was virtual. Supporting Covid patients in hospital, Imam Monawar had to resort to using phones or iPads to pray with the patients or to recite the Qur'an for them since he could not be at their bedside. He did the same for their families who could not visit their ailing relatives. Of his own experience, Imam Monawar said the past two years had been the hardest in his life, involving the greatest number of deaths he has dealt with. Islamic practice requires bodies to be interred as soon as possible after death, preferably within twenty-four hours if possible. Imam Monawar highlighted the exemplary working partnership in Oxfordshire between the Trust's doctors, bereavement department, the registrars, the coroner's office, the cemetery, local mosques and the Muslim funeral directors to ensure timely release of Muslim bodies. Issuing of the necessary paperwork was all done by email rather than in person.

Burial ablution

Imams and providers of funeral and burial services had to make decisions about whether or not to perform the religious requirement of body ablution (*ghusl*) during Covid. Some Imams and Muslim providers in the UK took the decision that in Covid circumstances the requirement of the *ghusl* could be waived and instead the body could be prayed over without the ritual washing or with dry ablution (*tayammum*) instead. In Oxford, Imam Monawar together with local Muslim funeral services and the hospital convened a webinar to discuss the matter of the *ghusl* with local Muslims. In consultation, it was decided that in Oxford the *ghusl* would be done. To cope with the extra work, the local Oxford services, Al Ansaar Funeral Services, trained volunteers who bravely stepped in to perform the ritual despite the potential risk to themselves. The volunteers donned full PPE to perform the obligatory ablution of the deceased. To reduce the emotional and mental impact of this highly demanding work, volunteers worked in rotation so that the same people were not doing the *ghusl* each time. Imam Monawar observed that he was heavily involved in supporting the bereaved, as there is not any specific faith-based community counselling support available yet in Oxford. He identified this local need for faith-based counselling support for the Muslim community in general, for volunteers and also for imams, as something to be addressed in the future.

Funerals

For family members who could not attend the funeral (*janāzah*) services of their deceased because they themselves were Covid positive, a YouTube channel was established so they could at least watch the funerals of their dear departed. Joint services for the customary fourth-day and fortieth-day prayers and Qur'an recitation were done by webinar for bereaved family and friends, with the words of the prayers and litanies up on screen, so they could pray altogether.

Covid has generated a huge sense of loss and grief. At the same time, as Imam Monawar noted, when people experience bereavement, they are driven to reflect on their own mortality, they see concretely the transience of this life on earth, and are led to reflect on the meaning of their lives and on how they are living. For instance, the value of family has come to the fore during the Covid crisis. Post-pandemic, people are even changing careers to find work which allows them to spend more time with their nearest and dearest. Families also stepped in to offer practical help to relatives badly affected by the pandemic. In the wake of loss of loved ones and amidst life-changing economic upheavals, a re-appreciation of family love and support is emerging.

'He has placed love and mercy between you' (Q. 30:21, *al-Rūm*, 'Byzantium').

Note

Qur'anic translations are the author's own and are rendered from the Standard Qur'anic Arabic text (Ḥafs ʿan ʿĀṣim recension), available in multiple formats. Transliteration is based on the Library of Congress system with modifications.

Acknowledgements

The author wishes to thank Imam Monawar Hussain (Muslim Chaplain, Oxford University Hospitals, NHS Foundation Trust) for sharing information about how the local Oxford Muslim community dealt with practicalities during the pandemic, in particular hospital and burial matters.

References

Burrell, David and Daher, Nazih (trans.) (1995). *Al-Ghazālī, the Ninety-Nine Beautiful Names of God* (*al-Maqṣad al-asnā fī sharḥ asmāʾ Allah al-ḥusnā*). Cambridge: Islamic Texts Society.

Campanini, Massimo (2012). 'The Muʿtazila in Islamic History and Thought'. *Religion Compass* 6 (1): 41–50.

Bearman, P. et al. (eds) (2012). '*Kasb*'. In *Encyclopaedia of Islam*, 2 ed., Leiden: Brill online. http://dx.doi.org/10.1163/1573-3912_ei2glos_SIM_gi_02109.

Felter, Claire (2021). *Will the World Ever Solve the Mystery of Covid-19's Origin?*. New York: Council on Foreign Relations.

Lowe, Derek (2022). 'The Origins of the Pandemic'. *Science*. 28 February. Accessible online at URL: https://www.science.org/content/blog-post/origins-pandemic.

Malik, Shoaib Ahmed (2021). 'Al-Ghazālī's Divine Command Theory'. *Journal of Religious Ethics* 49 (3): 546–76.

An-Nawawī, Yaḥyā ibn Sharaf (author of Arabic text), Ibrahim, Ezzedin and Johnson-Davies, Denys (trans.) (1997). *An-Nawawi's Forty Hadith*. Cambridge: Islamic Texts Society.
Watt, Montgomery W. (2012). 'Al-Ashʿarī, Abūʾl-Ḥasan'. In P. Bearman et al. eds, *Encyclopaedia of Islam*, 2 ed., Leiden: Brill online.

8

Turning to medicine is not turning away from God: Hindu resilience in a pandemic

Anantanand Rambachan

Faith and medicine

In his version of the Ramayana *(Sri Ramacaritamanasa)*, the life story of Rama who is venerated by millions of Hindus as God-incarnate *(avatar)*, the saintly poet Tulasidasa *(c.* fifteenth century CE) described a moment in the war between Rama and Ravana when Rama's younger brother, Lakshmana, was gravely wounded in the chest by a spear released by Ravana's son. Hanuman, the foremost among the servants of Rama, lifted the limp body of Lakshmana and brought him before Rama. They were all very distraught but knew that it was urgent to locate the most qualified physician, Sushena. Many among them believed that Rama was divine, but no one objected or argued; none condemned the efficacy of medical practice or called for a miraculous cure. No one saw the recourse to medical therapy as indicative of a lack of faith in the divine.

Hanuman found Sushena and returned with him to the battlefield. After he examined Lakshmana, Sushena recommended a herbal medication located on a distant mountain. The rest of the story is well known. Hanuman travelled to the mountain but was unable to identify the specific herb. Leaving no stone unturned, he lifted the mountain and returned to Sushena and Rama. Sushena prepared the medication, applied it and Lakshmana recovered from his wound.

The story of Hanuman finding the right physician and medicine illustrates many important aspects of the Hindu response to the pandemic. I am not aware of any divisions within Hindu communities centred on debates about the prioritizing of prayer or divine intervention over medical science. My local Hindu temple in Maple Grove, Minnesota, became a centre for vaccine dispensation and Hindus were encouraged to be vaccinated. Acharya Bhrigu Nath Shukla at the Sanatan Dharma Temple in Norwolk, California, exemplifies what is widespread among Hindu leaders. He refused to grant vaccine exemptions on religious grounds, encouraged vaccination and offered vaccinations at his temple (Medina 2021).

For Hindus, faith in the divine is not opposed to or tested by refusing medical treatment. Turning to medicine is not turning away from God. Hanuman's search for a medicinal cure for Lakshmana was done with the approval of the divine Rama to whom many miraculous actions are attributed in the Ramayana. God's purpose in the world is accomplished also through the efforts of compassionate human beings, in this case by those, like the physician Sushena, who labour in the cause of finding effective vaccines.

Tulasidasa, cited above, makes an important theological claim in the Ramayana about the nature of God and God's servants.

> God is the ocean; good people are the rain clouds.
> God is the sandal tree; good people are the winds.

(Tulasidasa 1984)

The oceans are our primary source of water; but rain clouds are nature's instruments for bringing to us the life-giving water of the ocean. The wood of the sandal tree emits a delicate and soothing fragrance; but the winds are necessary for bringing the fragrance to us. The rain clouds and the winds convey to us the blessings of the ocean and the sandal tree. In dealing with the challenges of Covid, Hindus see the blessings of God in the work of scientific researchers who, inspired by a passion for relieving suffering, left no stones unturned to find vaccines and curative therapies. Divine reality manifested in all who gave generously to others in the work of healing, comforting, supporting and accompanying.

Theodicy and Covid

As far as religious explanations for the occurrence of Covid are concerned, I did not see any significant theodicic speculations in Hindu communities. Popular theodicies such as the idea that God is using the pandemic to motivate human beings to change course, or that the pandemic is divine punishment for human transgression are not prominent in Hindu thought. Hindus affirm the doctrine of karma which emphasizes the relationship between human actions and their long-term consequences. Two of the well-known explanations for Covid, zoonotic transmission or the lab-leak hypothesis, are likely to be seen as pointing to human responsibility. In the case of zoonotic transmission, humans are responsible for habitat destruction and encroaching on the rapidly dwindling spaces of other species. We are also responsible for the unsanitary conditions and suffering of caged animals in wet markets. The lab-leak hypothesis also attributes responsibility to human beings. Both explanations grant primary responsibility to human beings for Covid and are consistent with the doctrine of karma. Covid does not diminish faith among Hindus because God is not held to be responsible. The Hindu response to Covid is pragmatic and empirical. It looks to rational causes and solutions, within the expansive framework of the doctrine of karma.

Domestic worship

The significant changes because of Covid, as far as Hindu practice is concerned, occurred with ritual worship. Hindu worship occurs primarily in homes and temples. Most Hindu homes have a special room or corner of a room set aside for the purpose of worship. In this space, the family's favourite iconic (*murti*) representations of God are kept. The *murti* is a visible reminder of God's presence and the home becomes a sacred space in which all aspects of life are centred on God. Worship in Hindu homes involves offerings of light, incense, flowers and food. Verses from sacred texts and the names of God are recited. Hindu domestic worship was not affected by Covid and enabled Hindus to continue with religious practices even when temples were closed. Although visiting and participating in temple worship are popular practices among Hindus, temple worship is not an obligatory religious requirement. The long tradition of domestic worship was a source of sustenance during Covid.

Temple worship

Hindu temples are regarded as special abodes of God. The living God is present in the temple in the form of the *murti*. *Murtis* that are made for temple worship undergo a series of consecratory rituals culminating in the establishment of the breath of life in the *murti* (*praṇapratiṣṭha*). The final step in this elaborate ritual occurs when the sacred artist completes his work by opening the eyes of the *murti*.

Once the *murti* is consecrated, it becomes a living embodiment of God who is honoured through the regular performance of hospitality rituals (*puja*). Worship starts in the quiet dawn with soft, solemn music and the recitation of sacred verses. This is followed by the ceremonial bath, after which the deity is anointed with sandal paste, dressed in royal robes and decked with ornaments and flowers. Worship ends with an elaborate evening light (*arati*) offering. All of these daily rituals, performed by temple priests, are obligatory and do not require the presence of congregants. The living deity cannot be ignored. Hindus visit the temple to witness these rituals at the end of which the priest gives to each attendee a portion of food offered to God (*prasada*), a few drops of the water used to wash the feet of the *murti* (*charanamrita*) and sandal paste, vermillion or ash on the forehead. The light that is waved before the icon is brought to each devotee and the *satari*, a gold or silver crown, with the imprint of the *murti*'s feet, is placed on the head of the worshipper as a mark of blessing.

For Hindus, the primary purpose of visiting a temple is to have *darshan* of the *murti*. The Sanskrit word, *darshan*, means 'seeing'. Hindus stand with reverential gazes before the *murti*, experiencing a profound sense of being in God's all-encompassing presence. *Darshan* is a dual mode of experience. While it is a profound sense of seeing God, it is, at the same time, a deep consciousness of being 'seen' by God. *Darshan* is meaningful in the context of the theology of the *murti* as living embodiment.

Temple worship is very sensual: one sees, hears, smells, touches and tastes. Every sense is activated in the experience of the divine. The closing of Hindu temples meant that such worship, in its immediacy, was not possible and this was a source of anguish for Hindus who frequent temples to witness and participate in rituals. They longed for the sanctified atmosphere of the temple and the physicality of worship. Online worship is not a substitute for these rich sensual ways of experiencing the divine.

For this chapter, I interviewed Sri Ronur Murali Bhattar, chief priest at the Hindu Temple in Maple Grove, Minnesota. He is a thirteenth-generation priest in his family and supervises a team of five priests at the temple. I also interviewed Pooja Bastodkar who served as President of the Executive Committee at the Hindu Society of Minnesota (2020–1) when the temple was challenged by Covid. Although both acknowledged the pain of worshippers who were unable to visit the temple, Muraliji (as he is affectionately called) explained that the daily round of temple rituals never ceased. These are obligatory once a *murti* is consecrated and do not require public presence or participation. These rituals were diligently performed each day by Muraliji and his priestly team. The fundamental purpose of these daily rituals, explained Muraliji, is the well-being of the world and so became even more significant in the circumstances of a pandemic. Bastodkar provided the priests, travelling back and forth to the temple, with letters explaining the nature of their work in the event that they were questioned by state authorities.

Temple leadership, Bastodkar explained, quickly recognized the religious dilemma of worshippers who were, at short notice, cut off from all temple activities because of the unprecedented closure of temple and the postponing of all festivals. In this respect, the obligatory nature of the temple rituals proved to be a great asset. To enable devotees to have *darshan* of the *murti*, and to witness the daily rituals, the temple authorities quickly arranged for online transmission of morning and evening rituals. In the words of Pooja Bastodkar, 'the concept of live-streaming events was creative and novel at the time, and thousands of devotees eagerly tuned in at specific times to watch our priests perform prayer rituals and recite age-old mantras' (Bastodkar 2021). The Hindu Temple in Maple Grove was one of the first in North America, said Bastodkar, to offer live-streaming of rituals and served as a resource and inspiration for other temples in this regard. The online experience of worship was, to say the least, different for Hindu devotees who regularly attended and participated in rituals, but it afforded continuity and ensured that they were not isolated. The large numbers testify to the value of the online availability of worship.

The establishment of a dedicated website for live-streaming at the Hindu Mandir in Minnesota allowed Hindus to interact with the priests and to personalize the rituals. Participation in a traditional Hindu worship ceremony requires the priest to know the names of the worshippers and their lineage. Hindus wishing to participate in temple worship were able to transmit this information to the priest who, with a laptop at hand, received it in real time. Devotees were able to hear their names included in the priest's prayer and to witness the ritual performed on the devotee's behalf. Computers took on a new role in the pandemic and became a medium for the experience of the sacred and communication with temple priests. Opportunities to participate in this way, explained Bastodkar, increased temple donations and helped to keep the institution solvent. Donation boxes (*hundis*), normally filled by temple visitors, stayed empty when the temple closed.

Ritual adaptation

Muraliji and his team of priests had to quickly adapt to novel ways of serving the Hindu community. Muraliji spoke of having to offer online instructions to family members to perform ceremonies for departed relatives, online marriage ceremonies and life-cycle rituals. Arrangements were made for individual online worship (*archana*) for those desiring such rituals and who were guided, step by step, by temple priests. Perhaps the most painful challenge for Muraliji and his team was offering support and religious services to Hindus in Minnesota with close family members who died from the virus in India. In the early months of the pandemic in India, the death rates were high, crematoriums were overwhelmed and bodies had to be quickly disposed in public spaces with minimum ritual. In some cases, the son or daughter qualified to perform the funeral and post-mortem rites (*shraddha*) resided in Minnesota. With closed borders, travel to India was not possible. For children in grief, unable to perform the final rites for a parent and without a deceased body, Muraliji used approved traditional alternatives. He guided such children through all the steps of a Hindu funeral ritual using an effigy of the parent made of grass. At the end, the effigy was cremated, and the ash immersed in flowing water as is the custom. Post-mortem rituals, required on specific days after death, were also performed by family members with the guidance of the priests. Such alternative rituals brought peace and healing to children in grief and enabled them to fulfil religious obligations to their parents. Rituals that evolved in ancient times to deal with the death of family members who undertook long and risky journeys of pilgrimage from which they may never return found new purpose under the conditions of a pandemic. Muraliji missed the company of devotees in front of the temple shrines, but his fellow priests were sources of support and ensured that life in the temple during the pandemic was not lonely.

The Hindu Temple in Maple Grove has now returned to normal functioning and worship is no longer live-streamed. The experience and success with live-streaming, however, Bastodkar told me, have generated discussions about the possibility of offering subscriptions for such an option. This option may be attractive to members of the community who have retired to other parts of the United States or for the elderly who are unable to travel to the temple. It may also enable Hindus in those parts of the United States without temples to experience and participate in temple rituals. For Bastodkar, the experience of physical isolation from the temple and from the company of other devotees has deepened her value for such association and made her more aware of its fragility. As a temple leader during a pandemic, she appreciates the need for prudence and good stewardship of resources to deal with crises of a similar nature in the future.

Hindu temples and communities demonstrated a remarkable resilience in facing the challenges of a global pandemic. The continuity of domestic worship, the obligatory nature of temple worship, the creative use of modern technology and the willingness of priests following ancient traditions to be flexible ensured continuity. The tradition's respect for science enabled temple leadership to strictly adhere to public health regulations and to meet the religious needs of the community in creative ways.

References

Bastodkar, Pooja (2021). 'The Sounds from Hundreds of Homes'. *Bearings Online*. 21 March 2021. Accessible online at URL: https://collegevilleinstitute.org/bearings/the-sounds-from-hundreds-of-homes/.

Medina, Vincent (2022). 'No Religious Exemption for Covid-19 Vaccine from Christian, Catholic Hindu leaders'. *Talon Marks*. 23 September 2021. Accessible online at URL: https://www.talonmarks.com/community/2021/09/23/no-religious-exemption-for-covid-19-vaccine-from-christian-catholic-hindu-leaders/.

Tulasidasa (1984). *Sri Ramacaritamanasa*. trans. R. C. Prasad. Delhi: Motilal Banarsidass.

9

Chanting, karma, love and Zoom: Hindu responses to a pandemic

Shaunaka Rishi Das and Utsa Bose

As the Coronavirus pandemic deepened its grip on the world, the questions of its causes, scientific, spiritual and karmic plagued the public imagination. Hinduism, too, grappled with these questions; and, in the absence of a central scriptural text, there arose a symphony of discourse.

Mother nature has a voice

One narrative around the Coronavirus pandemic was that it was a natural upshot of Environmental Hinduism. This was based on the argument that the pandemic was a force of natural balance. The earth, personified as the Goddess Bhumi, is known as one of the seven 'mothers' of the world; this opinion argued that the pandemic was a balancing act. On the surface, it was an act of painful loss – in the larger scope of things, however, this was a benefit. Mother nature was healing the world through a painful process of rebalance.

Another perspective was based on the law of karma. Karma is considered the natural principle of cause and effect. No act is seen as random; rather, it is an effect of another, older act, perhaps even from one's previous lives. The pandemic was an effect, then, of other causes. A form that this karmic argument took was that the pandemic was a reaction to global greed, one idea emphasizing greed leading to cruelty, the slaughter for profit of so many living beings, including animals, trees and aquatics – acts that are not now going unpunished. Expanding on Bhumi's act of balance, some supposed she was reacting to what was seen as our ever-increasing abuse of natural resources since the time of the Industrial Revolution. In response she sent one of her most insignificant soldiers, a virus, to show us how fragile our power is (and maybe who is our Mama) – effectively disrupting our economic systems, our social and political institutions, and our infrastructure – an eloquent display of her power.

Nestled in these narratives, however, was the tacit belief that the pandemic was a cause for global introspection; humans were not passive victims caught in the deluge, but active agents whose acts had accrued, and caused this calamity. There was hardly a voice that blamed God. It was understood that this was our mess, and the Supreme was the shelter, the source of strength to endure and the source of joy amidst distress.

I heard many voices, mainly online, explaining that material circumstances are cyclical; whatever starts must end. In the grander scope of this wheel of time many expressed the understanding that the pandemic was one in a series of small disruptions; moments like these had happened in the past and they would happen again. In the grand scope of things, this was merely a blip – this was no vision of Armageddon; the world would get up, dress up and show up again.

New pathways of practice and technoritualism

Hinduism has been surprisingly successful at adapting to new realities, and absorbing philosophies and religions, while concurrently representing age-old rituals, cultures and customs. Maybe predictably, then, Hindus innovated during the pandemic, specially within the realm of ritual and communication. It will be interesting to see how some of these adaptions will endure. Arguably, two of the most important rituals in Hinduism, maybe in any tradition, are the rituals associated with marriage and death. Both of these rites have great significance for Hindus, which anyone attending a three-day Hindu wedding will testify. There were many reported cases, in India, of family weddings going ahead during lockdown, with participants making a clear distinction between the need to isolate and the need to transcend Covid restrictions for a wedding. Marriage remained an exception to the rules of social quarantining. The idea of selective exception was even more apparent during the Kumbha Mela, the regular religious gathering of millions, who indeed turned up, not in spite of the pandemic but because of the pandemic. Surely, reported many participants, a pilgrimage, a duty of great spiritual importance transcends material inconvenience.

The pandemic, however, saw a shift in the relative emphasis given to religious rites at funerals. Journalist Natasha Mikles (2021) makes the argument that the surge in deaths due to the Covid pandemic led to a dearth of cremation grounds. This led to far-reaching ritual changes in the form of makeshift crematoriums being constructed in the parking lots of hospitals and in city parks. The pandemic also saw necessity resulting in young women partaking in the lighting of the funeral pyre, which was 'previously not permissible'. It also led to a disruption of the social culture of funerals. I led the service for an elderly Indian lady in London, attended by ten people, by restriction, but with more than six hundred attending online. It was painful to see the ten, mourning alone, not even being able to hug each other – a pathetic sight experienced by many, in many countries.

The pressure of newly recalibrated crematorium arrangements in India fell upon crematorium workers. As Saurabh Sharma's report in *Al Jazeera* suggests, with the worsening of the pandemic, Deen Dayal Verma, a crematorium worker in the city of Barabanki, was the only one who continued working in his particular crematorium. Arguing that the pandemic made 'family members refuse to touch the dead body' quite often, Verma stated that the fear of contagion led to many people viewing cremation ceremonies as a 'burden' and families just wanted to get rid of the dead bodies.

The story of Ankit Dwivendi, a twenty-three-year-old crematorium worker in Unnao, shows another shift in ritual practice. Ankit stated that the surge in cases had led to many Hindus wanting to 'bury their dead', when they could not 'get the cremation done as fast as possible'. The act of burying the dead is not unknown, but generally frowned upon in Hinduism. Dwivendi attributed this drastic change in ritual to both 'poverty, and the fear of Covid'. The article further stated:

[W]ith some priests afraid to oversee cremations due to the pandemic, the 23-year-old crematorium worker also performs their duties. Although he is not a priest and has received no training, it is Ankit who now quickly recites the funeral hymns.

(Sharma 2021)

The pandemic also saw changes in everyday religious practice. The panic, paranoia and alienness of the pandemic manifested in the form of new goddesses in the Hindu pantheon. The transference of an epidemic to a goddess is not new in Hinduism, and while worthy of mention, does not attract much attention among most Hindus. Previously there was Sitala, the goddess of smallpox, but now a new goddess manifest, varying from place to place. In Kerala, for example, as *The Hindu* reported, there was the case of Anilan, a resident of Kadakkal, who installed a form of a Corona Goddess (called 'Corona Devi') in his domestic shrine. He said that in 'Hindu mythology', 'God is omnipresent, and even exists in the virus', therefore 'worshipping a virus as devi is not an alien custom for us' (Staff Reporter 2020). It is interesting to note that the goddess here is not the destroyer of the disease – rather, it is a form of the omnipresent deity, thus meant to be propitiated. The Plague Mariamman Temple, in Coimbatore, traditionally famous for its deity of the Plague Goddess, also saw the addition of a 'Corona Devi' (Corona Goddess) form. As Kavita Muralidharan reported in the People's Archive of Rural India (PARI), the 'Corona Devi temple has not, for most of its existence, allowed worshippers to visit in person – because of lockdowns'. Another important addition was that it was not just the deity that was considered divine but pandemic protocols themselves. Further east, the city of Kolkata in West Bengal, where the cult of Kali reigns supreme, the pandemic saw the installation of a new form of the goddess, now wearing a mask for Covid awareness (News-18).

With goddesses changing form, forms of worship were altered too. In Anilan's case, for example, he argued that there would be no temple visitation and that the *prasadam* (blessed offerings) would be available to devotees via mail. Many temples across the Hindu world resorted to the use of Facebook livestreams, Zoom, email and messaging to continue ritual without human contact. This changed form of ritual, mediated by the use of new forms of technology – what could be termed 'technoritualism' – was another important innovation of the pandemic.

Hindus went online very quickly to fulfil every aspect of worship and practice. Communities and family groups were invited to more events, with more frequency than they had yet experienced. Congregations were strengthened and new communities of inquiry and worship manifest. In our Oxford Chaplaincy, where we would get about ten participants in our weekly study group, we now had fifty students on Zoom, from Canada to Australia, and that without any advertisement. Swamis and gurus from different Hindu denominations reported that they were much busier, and in contact with many more people during the pandemic. These e-gatherings helped allay panic as well as recuperating a sense of lost community. In the absence of social interaction, group calls with devotees across the world created new solidarities and possibilities of *sanga* – the association of the holy.

Appealing to God and science

An interesting outcome of the pandemic involves the improbable connections that were forged between Hinduism and science (as, I am sure, it was with every religion). The importance of religion in the pandemic cannot be overstated; The compounded effect of fear, death and a breakdown in socialization led to dilemmas that science is ill equipped to deal with effectively. During the early stages of the pandemic, in the absence of a vaccine and conclusive medical evidence, many Hindus had no other recourse but their poetry, chants, yogas, philosophies, pujas, sadhanas, prayers and art – and they were not lacking.

There were various instances of influential religious congregations helping the cause of scientific proliferation. In London, the Bochasanwasi Akshar Purushottam Swaminarayan Sanstha (BAPS) spread awareness about the PRINCIPLE trials, a UK-wide clinical study aimed at finding Covid-19 treatments for recovery at home. This collaboration, between the BAPS and the PRINCIPLE trials, led by the University of Oxford was largely fruitful in raising awareness and helped in 'reaching out to communities as widely as possible' (University of Oxford 2020). In India, the collaborations were also political, and not sectarian, as some may have expected. On 2 April 2020, Narendra Modi appealed to 'leaders of all religions, sects, caste, creeds and communities' (admin 2020) to help in the fight against the Coronavirus pandemic. Modi's appeal was significant because it delicately cradled the shifts which religions, and in our case Hinduism, witnessed because of the pandemic. Instead of relegating religious leaders during a 'scientific' crisis, his appeal signalled the importance of using the influence of religion, in a secular society, for the common good.

Any act of calamity and catastrophe is, for those of us who have had the privilege of survival, a time of introspection and learning. Amid a great flux in social order, the pandemic showed the constantly adaptive nature of Hindu practice. The crisis of the present, of course, often makes us look back at the past for traces, and echoes. In 1898, when the Third Bubonic Plague Pandemic struck the colonial capital, Calcutta, Swami Vivekananda issued a 'Plague Manifesto'. The contents of this small document mirror some concerns of our recent pandemic. The Swami stated that one should not fear the disease; that one should not, as he said, 'pay heed to rumours', and that vaccinations, insofar as they were becoming normalized, were not, as the rumours suggested, a forced endeavour. 'The British Government will not vaccinate anyone by force', he stated, 'Only those who are willing will be vaccinated' (Vivekananda 2022). In the absence of a known cure, he pushed for cleanliness, including internal cleanliness, stating finally that 'in order to remove the fear of the epidemic', one should sing the 'Nama Sankirtanam (i.e. chanting the names of God publicly) every evening, in every locality'.

He was here echoing an age-old custom, where chanting parties would manifest all over this region during an epidemic, chanting the name of Krishna. This practice was replicated during the current pandemic as well, with chanting parties appearing online with great regularly. A family *kirtan* gathering to which I was invited, and which would have attracted about twenty participants in person, hosted more than 340 on Zoom.

Vivekananda recognized that the importance of religion did not lie in the literal curing of the epidemic; rather, it lay in removing the 'fear of the epidemic', and in suggesting a spiritual alternative. Its potential lay in allaying panic, calming the frayed mind and focusing the heart on love of God. His suggested balance – of both vaccinating oneself and appealing to God – showed a continuity with Hindu responses more than a hundred years later. Sharing the grief of loss, and acknowledging personal disruption and trauma, that pandemic ended; so will this one, as will the next – a series of blips in the light of eternity.

References

admin (2020). 'PM Modi Appeals to Religious Leaders to Help in Fight against Coronavirus'. *ABP Live*. ABP. 2 April 2020. Accessible online at URL: https://news.abplive.com/videos/news/india-pm-modi-appeals-religious-leaders-to-help-in-fight-against-coronavirus-1187747.

Mikles, Natasha. 'Indians Are Forced to Change Rituals for Their Dead as COVID-19 Rages through Cities and Villages'. *The Conversation*, 4 May 2021. Accessible online at URL: https://theconversation.com/indians-are-forced-to-change-rituals-for-their-dead-as-covid-19-rages-through-cities-and-villages-160076.

Muralidharan, Kavita. 'In Coimbatore: Death, Disease and Divinity'. *PARI: People's Archive of Rural India*, 11 January 2022. Accessible online at URL: https://ruralindiaonline.org/or/articles/in-coimbatore-death-disease-and-divinity/.

News18 'Ma Kali Idol Wears Mask for Covid Awareness, Dakshineswar Temple in Kolkata Decked Up for Celebrations'. *News18*. 4 November 2021. Accessible online at URL: https://www.news18.com/photogallery/photogallery/ma-kali-idol-wears-mask-for-covid-awareness-dakshineswar-temple-in-kolkata-decked-up-for-celebrations-in-photos-4403255.html.

Sharma, Saurabh (2021). 'Tales from an Indian Crematorium'. *Al Jazeera*. 27 June 2021. Accessible online at URL: https://www.aljazeera.com/features/2021/6/27/india-covid-crisis-the-crematorium-workers.

Staff Reporter. 'Just One Devotee for 'Corona Devi'. *The Hindu*. 13 June 2020. Accessible online at URL: https://www.thehindu.com/news/national/kerala/just-one-devotee-for-corona-devi/article31816062.ece.

University of Oxford (2020). 'Britain's Most Influential Hindu Temple Spreads Awareness of the PRINCIPLE Trial among Indian Community'. University of Oxford, 22 October 2020. Accessible online at URL: https://www.ox.ac.uk/news/2020-10-22-britain-s-most-influential-hindu-temple-spreads-awareness-principle-trial-among.

Vivekananda, Swami. 'Swami Vivekananda's "Plague Manifesto"'. *Ramakrishna Mission Viayavada/Sitanagaram, Andhra Pradesh*. Accessible online at URL: https://www.rkmissionvijayawada.org/swamijis-plague-manifesto/.

10

The Buddha's prescription for the world: How people used Buddhism to cope with the pandemic

Bogodá Seelawimala

During the Covid epidemic monks had nobody to address, and only empty seats in front of them. Now after such a long time we have opened our doors and can begin to understand how Buddhism helped to the people to face this unprecedented situation.

The Buddha: Master of medicine

The Buddha was a great compassionate doctor and pointed out that disease is an inevitable part of our lives. In the very first discourse, the Buddha pointed out that disease is a signpost of our suffering (*vyadipi dukkha*). The Buddha explained there are two types of diseases: physical disease (*kayika roga*) and mental disease (*cetasika roga*). For mental health, the Buddha's teachings have been compared to medicine, and the Buddha introduced as a peerless physician (*bhisakko*), the supreme surgeon (*sallakatto anuttaro*) (*Ittivutaka* 100). Some statues of the Buddha's show him holding a bowl in his hand, symbolizing a container of medicine. In Far Eastern countries such as Japan, Korea and China where Mahayana Buddhism is widely practised the concept of the 'medicine Buddha' and many related icons are popular. These statues demonstrate the Buddha as a teacher of medicine (*bhaisajja guru*), and to illuminate that the main purpose of the Buddha's appearance was to convince us of universal suffering (*dukkha*) and the cessation of suffering (*nirodha*). In one discourse there are shown forty-four diseases of the mind, and the Buddha has prescribed treatments for such sicknesses. In the *Sallekha Sutta*, he says, 'Bhikkhus, there is no medicine better than Dhamma (doctrine), which is comparable to any medicine in the world.'

The concept of the Buddha as a teacher of medicine has been articulated in the story of Kisagotami. The story tells us that when her young child had died, she refused to believe he was dead. Asking many people in vain for medicine that would revive the child, she was finally directed to the Buddha. When she told him her story, the Buddha addressed her very kindly, 'Sister I can help you.' He offered to provide medicine for the child, but said he would need some mustard seed – the cheapest Indian spice – obtained from a family in which no one had ever died. She went from house to house asking for mustard seed, but when she asked if anyone had died in the family, the universal response was always, yes, and they told many stories of deaths of relatives, families, father, mother and children. The message sunk in: Death is universal. She left her child's body at a charnel ground. The Buddha's way of convincing her was like medicine, and it healed her mind, and she returned to the Buddha and asked to be ordained as a nun (Sayadaw 2011:58).

Under the modern concept of well-being, in the field of medicine, there are several aspects to consider: physical, mental, spiritual, social, environmental and economic, and Covid has challenged all these aspects of life. In Buddhist teachings, the maintenance of all these aspects has been recommended as the way to achieve a peaceful, successful and happy life. All can be summarized under the Buddha's saying, 'Health is the greatest gift, contentment is the greatest wealth, a trusted friend is the best relative, nirvana is the greatest bliss' (*Dhammapada* 204).

When we look at the practices and principles of Buddhists, observers start their spiritual journey by taking refuge in the Buddha, Dhamma and Sangha (the Buddha, his teaching and the monastic community). The Buddha advised; 'I also say unto you O Monks – if any fear, terror or hair standing-on-end should arise in you, ... then think only of me.' 'Monks, if you think of me, any fear, terror, or standing of hair-on-end, that may arise in you, passes away.' 'If you fail to think of me, then think of the Dhamma, if you fail to think of the Dhamma, then think of the Sangha' (Piyadassi 2018). But here, more relevant, is the objective to discover how Buddhism helped us to face the fear caused by the Covid pandemic. During the pandemic, the Buddhist community followed Buddhist practice as medicine for health security. They practised the three key aspects of Buddhism: listening to sermons, meditation and listening to chanting.

Listening to sermons

Listening to sermons and Dhamma talks was widely used during the period of the pandemic. The Buddha identified six qualities of the Dhamma: being well proclaimed by the Buddha, self-realized, bearing immediate fruit, inviting investigation, leading on to Enlightenment (nirvana). The main purpose of the Dhamma, as mentioned above, is the cessation of suffering.

The Buddha once, when crossing a forest, collected some leaves, put them on his palm and asked the monks, 'Are the leaves on my palm less or more than the leaves in the forest?' The monks answered, 'The leaves on the palm are very little'. The Buddha replied, 'Certainly, I teach you about suffering and cessation of suffering, although I know much more than suffering, likewise the other leaves are not conducive to cessation of suffering' (*Simsapa Sutta* 56:31).

Buddhism does not promise answers to all the metaphysical questions which the people asked. For instance, if a person was shot by a poisonous arrow and said, 'I won't allow for this arrow to be taken from my body until someone answers: What kind of bow was I was shot with? What is the person's caste? What is his name and family?, What is the person's colour? Is he tall, short or medium? What kind of bow string was used? With what kind of material was the point of the arrow made? Without knowing any of these things I will not allow this arrow to be removed' – The Buddha said the person would die with these unanswered questions. The most important task is taking the arrow from the body. Likewise, the Buddha pointed out the spiritual urgency for overcoming suffering (Woodward [1925] 1951: 305–7). If we get sick, it is wise to take most urgent and direct action. Therefore, if the answers are beneficial and conducive to spiritual development or useful for a successful home life, the Buddha would answer such questions.

Meditation

Buddhism does not advise people to follow extremes; it is a middle path (*majjima patipada*). The four noble truths – suffering, the cause of suffering, cessation of suffering and the path to the cessation of suffering – are at the heart of his teaching which is based on following the middle path – so, during the pandemic we had good chance to learn the Dhamma, following a path between mixing in crowds and suffering lonely isolation. The second area of the practice is meditation. For meditation practice, separation from crowds is recommended in the discourses. This separation and other activities are called *kaya viveka*. A quiet area, a grove or a forest are congenial for practice. Such an environment automatically appeared due to the restrictions of social distancing. During the pandemic, we continued our mediation classes online, as we were conscious that, due to the restrictions of social distancing, people would experience loneliness, fear, anxiety and even depression. In this connection, many researchers like Nicole Valtorta of Newcastle University pointed out that 'Lacking encouragement from family or friends, those who are lonely, may slide into unhealthy habits', adding, 'In addition, loneliness has been found to raise levels of stress, impede sleep and, in turn, harm the body. Loneliness can also augment depression or anxiety' (Valtorta et al 2015).

The Buddha said, 'oneself, indeed, is one's own saviour, for what other saviour would there be? With oneself well-controlled, one obtains a saviour difficult to find' (Dhammapada 160). We have to learn to take care of ourselves. The practice of meditation is a highly beneficial method to transform the mind. In Buddhism, meditation is called bhavana, which means mental development or cultivation. In Buddhism, meditation has two qualities: tranquillity (Samatha) and Insight (Vipassana), based on mindfulness, which are at the heart of the Buddhist path. Tranquillity mediation develops a wholesome, peaceful state of the mind. The most recommended object to focus on during mediation is breathing. When one experiences peace with deep tranquillity of the mind, it is easier to overcome stress and negativities such as desire, ill-will, sloth, torpor, restlessness, worry, doubt, loneliness and anxiety. A half-hour period of simple practice can bring about a peaceful state of mind, with a deep feeling of relaxation.

Vipassana (insight) meditation

Mainly, the Sathipatthana Sutta gives details of mindfulness practice (Maha Satipatthana Sutta: 335–50). As we deepen our concentration then we practise Vipassana. 'Vi' means special and 'passana' seeing – a way of 'seeing things as they truly are'. The mindfulness techniques are a guide to awaken us from moment to moment, always experiencing non-judgemental awareness, in the present moment. In practice, we can watch the thoughts passing through our mind; however, in the practice of Vipassana, by simply watching, we experience the nature of impermanence through ever-changing phenomena; everything we experience within the mind and body complex clearly sharpens our cognitive ability. In modern days, mindfulness practice is used widely as a stress reduction method (UMass Mental Health 2022).

We can understand that feeling, sensations, emotions, moods, images and thoughts arise and pass away; we do not identify with them as Self, as Mine. Thoughts such as worry and stress are impermanent, we do not regard them as *my* worry or *my* stress. They are just passing states of mind. We note them and let them go. Psychologists have pointed out these self-centred, negative thought processes are the cause of depression. In this field, lots of research has been done. According to Professor Zindel Segal (2018), who introduced Mindfulness Base on Cognitive Therapy (MBCT), generating negative thought processes based on self-centeredness is one of the main reasons for depression. In Buddhism these diversified thought processes are called *papanca* (see Nanananada [1971] (1997)). The Buddha recommended wise consideration (*yoniso manasikara*) as a good technique to eliminate the negative thought process from the moment they start, and to stop them from preoccupying the mind. So, the practice of mindfulness stops the mind going astray and aims to guide our mind in the right direction.

Metta Bhavana Meditation, or Meditation on Loving Kindness, is based on the *Metta Sutta*, a discourse which especially highlights this quality. This is one particular kind of meditation which could be regarded as a form of prayer. Metta is unconditional goodwill towards all beings, wishing them to be happy and free from suffering, starting with oneself; with practice, this enables us to radiate pure thoughts in an ever-widening circle, so that all beings are embraced without exception or limitation. This practice is normally done by repeating simple phrases, such as 'May I be free from anger and ill-will; may I be free from fear and anxiety; may I be free from pain and suffering; may I be happy and peaceful.' These words are then repeated in a variety of ways, replacing the word 'I' with 'beings in this hall', 'beings in this town', 'beings in this country', 'beings in the world', 'beings in the universe' and more. This sending of loving-kindness in every direction, to all beings without exception, can be regarded as a form of prayer in which, though there is no calling on a deity, the practitioner is generating potent forces within themselves which purifies their mind of negative qualities such as anger, ill-will and resentment.

These three types – tranquillity, mindfulness and loving kindness meditation practice – are widely used and are conducive to transforming our minds from loneliness and other negative attitudes and feelings.

Paritta chanting

During the time of the pandemic, monks in all the monasteries practised chanting, wishing to eliminate the epidemic and alleviate the harm it was causing to society. Here in our monastery, in the mornings, and especially in the evenings, all the monks gave guided meditation and chanted online via Facebook, Zoom and YouTube to give blessings to the people. Lots of people joined our chanting ceremony and allocated this period in their day to listen to our chanting.

Several chaplaincy services in hospitals requested our help for Buddhist patients who were in a very severe condition, being positive with Covid. As we too were vulnerable, unable to approach directly, on such occasions we asked them to make video calls and we provided counselling and chanting, and we distributed CDs of chanting to several hospitals. In our chanting we never forget to choose the jewel discourse (*Ratana Sutta*), which refers to the qualities of the Buddha, Dhamma and Sangha. For chanting, the Ratana Sutta explains the qualities of the Buddha, Dhamma and Sangha. Each stanza ends by the affirmation, 'May there be happiness.' There is a story behind this discourse. When the Buddha was living in the city of Vishala, there was an epidemic similar to the recent pandemic. Many people lost their lives. The story goes that people in the city were suffering, overwhelmed by the triple fear of famine, disease and evil spirits. Many dead bodies lay in the streets and everyone else was helpless. People had performed many rituals and sacrifices to overcome the situation. The Buddha was invited to visit the city and went there with his attendant monk, Ananda, and chanted the Ratana Sutta. After he performed his chanting, there was a downpour – and the rain marked the end of triple fear.

In the Buddha's time, when monks became sick, the Buddha asked other monks to chant the *Bojjhanga Paritta*. Bojjhanga, means 'factors of enlightenment'. There are seven factors in the Buddhist Scriptures, namely Mindfulness (*sati*), reflection on the Dhamma (*dhammavicaya*), Effort (*viriya*), Rapture (*piti*), Tranquillity (*passaddhi*), Concentration (*samadhi*), and Equanimity (*upekkha*). Chanting this scripture helped the monks to heal, as they had participated in the chanting with their fellow monks on many occasions. The Buddha's treatment for a sick person was to treat the mind. As pointed out earlier, his teachings are like medicine (*dhammosadha*). Whoever chants finds that their motivation is led by loving kindness (*metta*) and compassion (*karuna*). Buddhist people believe chanting has a healing power and it is a great blessing for good health. We mainly practised *paritta* chanting for patients during the pandemic.

Consumption

Why Covid has caused such devastation is a very hard question to answer. However, in Buddhism several reasons are given for the manifestation of illness, and the pandemic taught us one simple lesson: improper consumption habits (*visama-parihārajā-ābādhā*) not only cause illnesses, and a simple virus can obliterate a considerable proportion of humanity.

Improper consumption is rooted in greed and ignorance and inevitably results in ill-health. The Buddha often recommended moderation in food (*bhojane matthagnu*) to his disciples. The Buddha included this practice in the moral codes (*patimokkha*) for the monks. Many Buddhists are vegetarian, being mindful of the consumption of food and their day-to-day activities. According to our personal experiences, these practices bear very positive results. In recent times people, especially the younger generations, have developed a greater awareness of their food, and also clothes and social relationships; society is, more and more, exercising 'carefulness' which is akin to mindfulness.

Charity (*dana*) means giving useful material or spiritual guidance to people in need, without expecting anything in return, not even a word of thanks. For monks, giving dhamma talks (*dhamma dana*) which are food for the mind; and encouraging fearlessness is also a *dana* which is called *abhayadana*. Compassion leads to the practice of welfare activities, and actively seeking out victims experiencing tragic events. When we practice generosity, we realize that we are all inter-connected, regardless of religious, cultural, national or ethnic boundaries.

Communication

As mentioned earlier, modern communication systems are highly developed and we were able to see each other on screen, although this is not the same as face-to-face interaction. We had to face the challenge with a positive response. Physical presence of people in our lives cannot be bettered; it is important in our social relationships. Nonetheless, due to the progress of new communication facilities like Zoom, YouTube, Facebook and other online capabilities, all our official or institutional activities could be fulfilled. Religious organizations changed and adapted with the development of these communication systems; more people accrued greater knowledge by listening to talks and joining dialogues and conferences. The horizon of wisdom widened with these new methods of communication. Certainly, this period marks the beginning of a new form of civilization for humankind.

Buddhist chanting, meditation and dhamma talks are now global, thanks to modern forms of communication. This practical, helpful 'medicine' is a sort of nutrition for the mind, greatly helping to overcome negative emotions such as fear, anxiety, loneliness, depression and hopelessness, engendering a feeling of calm to our physical being and bringing about much-needed peace to our restless spirits.

References

Dhammapada, trans. Daw Mya Tin (1986). Rangoon: Tipitaka Burma Association. Accessible online at URL: https://www.tipitaka.net/tipitaka/dhp/index.php.

Itivuttaka: The Group of Ones, trans. John D. Ireland (2013). Access to Insight (BCBS Edition). Accessible online at URL: http://www.accesstoinsight.org/tipitaka/kn/iti/iti.1.024-027.irel.html.

Maha Satipatthana Sutta, in Walshe, Maurice (trans.) (2005), *Digha Nikaya*. Somerville, MI: Wisdom Publications.

Metta Sutta, Sutta Nipata, trans. H. Saddhatissa (1985). London: Curzon Press.

Nanananda, Bhikkhu ([1971] 1997), *Concept and Reality in Early Buddhist Thought*. Kandy: Buddhist Publication Society.

Piyadassi, Thera, (trans.) (2018). *Dhajagga Sutta, The Book of Protection*. Accessible online at URL: https://www.buddhanet.net/e-learning/buddhism/bp_sut11.htm.

Sallekha Sutta. Accessible online at URL: https://www.accesstoinsight.org/tipitaka/mn/mn.008.nypo.html.

Sayadaw, Mahasi (2011). *A Discourse on the Sallekha Sutta*. Rangoon: Buddha Sāsanānuggaha Organization.

Segal, Zindel, Mark Williams, and John Teasdale (2018). *Mindfulness-Based Cognitive Therapy for Depression*. New York: Guildford.

Sinsapa Sutta, SN. 56.32 in *Samyutta Nikaya*, trans. Bhikkhu Bodhi (2003), *Connected Discourses of the Buddha*, Boston: Wisdom Publications.

Sutta Nipata, trans. H. Saddhatissa (1985). London: Curzon Press.

UMass Memorial Health (2022). 'Everyone Experiences Stress. It's a Part of the Human Experience.' Accessible online at URL: www.ummhealth.org/center-mindfulness.

Valtorta, Nicole K. et al. (2015). Loneliness, Social Isolation and Social Relationships: What Are We Measuring? A Novel Framework for Classifying and Comparing Tools. *BMJ Open* 2016;6:4. DOI:10.1136/bmjopen-2015-010799. Accessible online at URL: http://orcid.org/0000-0002-9694-7965.

Woodward, F. L. (ed.) ([1925]1951). *Some Sayings of the Buddha*. London: Oxford University Press.

11

Covid and Theravada Buddhism

Peter Harvey

Making sense of Covid

For Buddhists, being born as a human being is seen as a fortunate rebirth, a product of past good karma, and with the opportunity for ethical and spiritual progress that may lead either to one's next life being as a human or in one of the long-lasting but non-eternal heavens, or to transcending all rebirths by attaining nirvana (liberation). Illness of various forms is seen as an inevitable aspect of living in a changing, impermanent world of many interacting conditions: part of the 'ageing, sickness and death' that all beings, including humans, are subject to. For Buddhists, being reminded of these realities and calmly reflecting on them can have a beneficial meditative effect (Harvey 2015).

Life is acknowledged to involve various forms of *dukkha*: mental and physical pains, especially those arising from clinging desire, and from aversion. Illness also increases as we age, and the complex system of the body-mind starts to develop faults. Or illness can arise from a variety of external causes, including catching a virus. The *Girimānanda Sutta* says that bodily afflictions include:

> illnesses originating from bile, phlegm, wind, or a combination of these; illnesses produced by seasonal change; illnesses produced by careless behaviour; illnesses produced by exertion; or illnesses produced as a result of karma (*kamma-vipa-ka-ni-jā*).

> (Bodhi 2012: 1411–15)

The *Sivaka Sutta* (Bodhi 2005, 1278–79) lists these as the various causes of (unpleasant) feelings and emphasizes that it is *incorrect* to say, 'Whatever this person experiences, whether pleasant or painful or neither painful nor pleasant, all that is due to what was done earlier.'

This passage is discussed in the *Milinda-pañha* (Horner 1969: 187–92), where King Milinda is described as wrongly thinking that 'all that is experienced is rooted in karma'. The monk Nāgasena points out the various causes of feelings, as above, and denies that karma underlies them all. Bodily winds, for example, can arise from a number of physical causes, though *some* do also arise due to past karma. On feelings in general, he says 'small is what is born of the maturing of karma, greater is the remainder' (Horner 1969: 135). Of course, to suffer from human illnesses, one needs to be reborn a human, and have the karma for this, so in a general sense, all illnesses have some karmic input. And genetic illnesses must be seen by a Buddhist as specifically due to karma, as one gets one's genes from one's parents but who one's parents are is a result of one's past karma.

So, the fact that someone catches a virus, or becomes very ill or dies from it, may be due to their past karma, or it may not be. There may be a karmic component if, for example, one is very careless as regards one's hygiene or mask-wearing, especially if one believes that Covid-19 is a 'hoax' and does not take the opportunity to be vaccinated against it. As regards the cause for the Covid-19 starting to spread among humans, this seems to have been due to humans encroaching on more of nature and eating wild infected creatures, thus being part of human over-exploitation of nature. Of course, the more such behaviour is accepted and spreads, the more people behave in bad ways and the risk of new viruses spreading to humans increases.

Our shared world

The fact that people around the world are having a shared experience of facing the virus has had a positive effect of drawing us all together in a shared experience. In our own countries, appreciation and gratitude for health workers has also been strengthened as we acknowledge how they help us all in this difficult time. Of course, the reduction of human activities in lockdowns has also allowed animals to visit our human world more – such as the hare that I saw in my garden one morning – so we have sometimes felt closer to nature, in a non-exploitative way.

In Sri Lanka also, during long spells of strict lockdown, people began to appreciate the positive impact on nature of these. The free movements of birds and animals, and the flowers blooming and other foliage in otherwise-busy cities, never previously noticed in the mad office rush, were often highlighted in the media. And reduction of the air pollution levels was also appreciated. Often heard was the suggestion that Covid may in fact be a blessing in disguise as a much-needed lesson from the universe to put our value system back on track.

Helpful Buddhist practices

Mindfulness and heedfulness are qualities emphasized by Buddhism, so this has helped us be careful of what we touch, as a kind of mindfulness of the body practice. Mindfulness of breathing has also aided being mindful of the air we share with those around us; indeed, wearing a mask has sometimes helped one be more mindful of one's breathing! Similarly, mindfulness has also helped in being more aware of the space round us, in which we and others move. Concentration on such things as breathing, or qualities of the Buddha, his teachings and the spiritual community of course aids calm, which is always beneficial, but especially in these times, which can bring anxiety. Chanting also has a calming effect on the body and mind. And patience and equanimity can also help us deal with the long haul of repeated lockdowns. We can also draw on *mettā* and *karuṇā*, lovingkindness and compassion, to encourage us to take care of the health of family members, friends and others we interact with and often depend on – as well as ourselves. Also, to watch out for anger at those seemingly careless of the health of others.

Some Buddhist chants known as *paritta* or *pirit*s are specifically seen as having a protective effect (Harvey 1993). How might they be seen to work? Firstly, to chant or listen to a *paritta* is soothing and leads to self-confidence and a calm, pure mind, due to both its sound quality and meaning. As the mind is in a healthier state, this may cure psychosomatic illnesses, strengthen the immune system, and make a person more alert and better at avoiding the dangers of life. Secondly, chanting a *paritta,* especially one which expresses lovingkindness to all beings, may calm down a hostile person, animal or ghost, making them more well-disposed towards the chanter and listeners. Thirdly, as well as generating new *puñña* – 'merit', good karma, or karmic fruitfulness – *paritta*-chanting may stimulate past karmic fruitfulness into bringing some of its fruits immediately. Fourthly, chanting or listening to a *paritta* is thought to please those gods who are devotees of the Buddha, so that they offer what protection and assistance it is in their power to give. Finally, the spiritual power of the Buddha, and of the truth he expressed, is seen as continuing in his words, with its beneficial influence being liberated when these are devoutly chanted.

As I see things, the protective power of *paritta*s largely comes from the good states of mind they help induce, and the harmonious energy that these and the chant infuse through the body. I would certainly not see *paritta*s as preventing one catching the virus, except through helping one be more careful. Nor would they necessarily prevent serious illness, or even death, from the virus. However, they may well help strengthen a person's general level of health and so help their body fight the virus and lessen its effects, especially if this in addition to having been vaccinated. Of course, our heedfulness as regards the threat from the virus also needs to be exercised in Buddhist contexts. Communal chanting, even of *paritta*s, could spread the virus, unless it is done outdoors, and with good spacing between people. One can of course chant them oneself in the home. Offering of *dāna* (alms-food and other offerings) to monks would also need to be done very carefully, so as not to transmit the virus.

The effects of Covid lockdowns

The lockdowns of course meant that in-person group meetings stopped. However, it meant that we were all introduced to Zoom (or similar ways of meeting through online services such as Facebook). While some do not like using Zoom, and such meetings do not give the full aspects found in in-person meetings, I feel they give 90 per cent of this. What is more, they have enabled meetings including people from around the UK and also beyond – Europe, North America, South Africa and sometimes Asia, dependent on time-zone differences. In this way, the world has shrunk in apparent size, as we have become more connected. This has enabled a great opening up of meditation teaching to those who could not normally access it or access particular forms of it.

Using Zoom for teaching meditation, and practising together, has been found to be very effective, as one still gets facial expressions, gestures and tones of voice, and good discussions. Like in-person meetings, it is still 'face to face', but in two rather than three dimensions. Meditation meetings have not just been weekly ones for an hour or two, but in some cases online meditation days. One key difference is as regards chanting. Chanting together produced a cacophony, due to time-lags, so it has to be done with a chant leader and everyone else on 'mute'. That said, different chants can be led by different people in a meeting.

Zoom has also facilitated online talks, which are then recorded and placed on a website or YouTube. As one does not need to travel to such events, this has of course saved on time, increased attendance and saved on our carbon footprints. Zoom has also made possible small groups of people from scattered locations to engage in study groups and working together in exploring some aspect of Buddhist teaching in relation to participants' everyday lives. Zoom and Skype or Face-time have also been used for one-to-one meetings between a meditation teacher and a meditator reporting on how their meditation is going. This was previously only done in person, but can now be done online with distant meditators.

As lockdown restrictions lessened, hybrid meetings have developed, with a small group of people meeting in-person, and others 'present' through Zoom. This has included meetings for funerals. Those with technical expertise have proved very useful for such hybrid meetings. Now lockdowns have ended, at least in the UK, online meetings will continue alongside in-person and hybrid meetings.

Buddhism in Asia

The above mainly concerns Western Buddhists, but what of Buddhists in Asia? In Thailand, for example, Buddhism is very social and revolves around religious and ritual acts that people conduct together, as families, as friends, as colleagues. There are shared gatherings for merit-making, *dāna,* celebrations, and funerals. Public activities are usually held in wide, high-ceilinged structures with plenty of room and good circulation of air. These features mean that the daily life of religion can continue, everyone carefully wearing masks and cautiously keeping space around them. Still, large gatherings do not take place, and the communal lay eating after the *dāna* is reduced or stopped. Many people do not go out at all, including to temples, if travel on public transport would be needed for this. Monks continue with their morning alms-rounds, wearing masks and keeping distance. People send donations for various reasons by electronic transfers, for example, to their village or regular temple. There are online functions and sermons by Zoom.

In Sri Lanka, the sense of impermanence, often limited to words, hit the greater majority of the Buddhists in its true sense. The quarantine processes and lockdowns were very strictly implemented, particularly in the first two rounds of the pandemic. When a family member was diagnosed Covid-positive and was taken in an ambulance to a quarantine centre, often with no symptoms or mild symptoms, people understood that they might not see their loved one again, though they might be perfectly healthy at the time of leaving the house. This was because in the event of death, no normal funerals were allowed: relatives or friends in full protective gear were only allowed to watch from afar, the coffin being brought and placed in the cremation chamber.

The usual religious ceremonies conducted by the side of the coffin, and the presence of monks, were not allowed. This was a quite a contrast to the usual practice in Sri Lanka, where the body is usually brought home at least for 24 hours with the coffin kept open throughout.

That said, funerals being simpler and more austere were generally appreciated as more in line with central Buddhist values. The pomp and pageantry often associated with a funeral irrespective of income level, with costly coffins, funerals dragging on for days and elaborate religious ceremonies to bestow merit on the departed were curtailed. There were coffins offered in the market made of board that, though looking elegant, were hitherto unthinkable. Similarly, weddings and corporate events which are also a show of wealth even amongst the not-so-rich have been curtailed in general. The curtailing of religious ceremonies in temples such as the *kathina* donation ceremonies, whose costs often run into millions of rupees (defying the spirit of the event), is conspicuous (1 million Sri Lankan rupees = 3,635 UK pounds).

Events on Zoom have become the order of the day for people of all walks of life and all age groups: even those who were hitherto not connected on the internet are seen engaging intensely. These have included sessions of meditation, discussions, readings of discourses of the Buddha and retreats. Full-day religious programmes for the laity have also gone online from temples, on the four days a lunar month on which people often visit temples and take extra precepts of ethical discipline, and include a mix of sermons, discussions and meditation.

One meditator reported that she has been participating in an online group that was 'so intense that, at the height of the pandemic, when the rest of the world was gripped by fear and anxiety, we often seemed to forget that there was a problem. The intensity was such that this group ... completed a word to word reading and discussion of many long texts', in Pali with explanations by the leading monk in Sinhala and questions and answers. Even formal counselling with Buddhist insights, for both individuals and groups, was offered on Zoom by the Damrivi Foundation.

As seen in all disaster situations, both monks and lay people were engaged in organizing the collection and distribution of food and other essentials to the needy, particularly to the daily wage earners who are deprived during lockdowns. During the height of the pandemic, the temples had texts such as the *Ratana Sutta* (a *paritta* text to help with illness), *Girimānanda Sutta* (Bodhi 2012: 1411–15) and *Bojjhaṅga Sutta* (Bodhi 2005: 1580–81), blasting through the loudspeakers at least twice a day. People in general took to regular chanting seriously as a protective measure. The moment travel restrictions were lifted, temples were seen attracting hundreds of people, particularly even when a new wave of the virus arrived: thousands flock for religious observances in places like Ruwanweliseya-Anuradhapura, Kelaniya and Sri Maha Bodhi Tree. The greater majority seemed to have felt starved of their religious observances during lockdown situations and travel restrictions, so much so they are seen bringing newborn babies and the feeble elderly irrespective of the very high risks.

References

Aṅguttara Nikāya, (trans.) Bhikkhu Bodhi, *The Numerical Discourses of the Buddha*. Wisdom, 2012.

Harvey, P. (1993). 'The Dynamics of Paritta Chanting in Southern Buddhism'. in K. Werner, ed., *Love Divine: Studies in Bhakti and Devotional Mysticism,* Richmond: Curzon Press, 53–84: https://www.academia.edu/24977532/The_Dynamics_of_Paritta_Chanting_in_Southern_Buddhism

Harvey, P. (2015). 'Introductory Reflections on Buddhism and Healing', *Buddhist Studies Review*, 32 (1): 13–18. https://journal.equinoxpub.com/BSR/article/view/9003/10476

Horner, I. B. (1969). *Milinda's Questions,* vol. I, London: Luzac & Co.

Saṁyutta Nikāya, (trans.) Bhikkhu Bodhi, *The Connected Discourses of the Buddha*. Wisdom, 2005.

To hear some *parittas*

– The Samatha Trust chanting: http://www.samatha.org/chants – Mettasutta
– Buddhanet chanting files: http://www.buddhanet.net/audio-chant.htm – Ratana Sutta

The author would like to express his thanks to Yuki Sirimane of Sri Lanka, Peter Skilling of Thailand, and people of Buddhist groups in York.

12

Fostering everyday culture at Shinto shrines under Covid

Taishi Kato

In Shinto, the world is thought to be composed of the workings of eight million *kami* (deities). The workings of these *kami* are considered to be beyond the reach of human manipulation and control. The most famous definition of *kami* in Japan was given by the Japanese scholar Motoori Norinaga in the Edo period (1603–1868).

Any form of beings whatsoever which possesses some unique and eminent quality, and is awe-inspiring, may be called *Kami*. 'Eminent' does not refer simply to nobility, goodness or special merit. Evil things or strange things, if they are extraordinarily awe-inspiring, may also be referred to as *Kami* (Hardacre 2017: 329).

Both good and evil workings exist for human beings. Considering *kami*'s work in the current pandemic situation, it is believed that the pestilence epidemic is also *kami*'s work and that it is *kami*'s work to quell it.

Looking back on Japanese history, people have always prayed to *kami* for the calming of epidemics. In an age when science and medicine were still underdeveloped, this wish would have been even more earnest. In Shinto, it has been believed that while *kami* is the one who calms the epidemic, *kami* is also the one who spreads the epidemic. The *kami* who spread the disease was called the *kami* of pestilence, and people tried to prevent the spread of the epidemic by worshipping and sometimes exorcising the *kami* in order to calm the epidemic. For example, one of the most feared diseases in Japan since ancient times was smallpox. People worshipped the disease as '*kami* of an epidemic' and held events such as 'sending off pemphigus *kami*' to drive them out of the village to avoid contracting pemphigus.

This pandemic is also an epidemic of pestilence, and prayers are being offered at Shinto shrines across the country to quell the pestilence through a ritual called 'The New Coronavirus Pandemic Calm Down Prayer'. The wish to quell the epidemic has been handed down to the present in the form of Shinto ceremonies.

Hare and Ke

The act of praying to quell the epidemic has not changed over time, but the Corona has affected both the shrine and the way people live their lives. Yanagita (1969) proposed that Japanese people's lives could be analysed from the perspective of time and space, '*hare* and *ke*'. '*Hare* and *Ke*' is a concept of time and space defined by Yanagita in the 1930s to describe a traditional view of the world. '*Hare*' is a word for special days and places used for celebratory events, and '*Ke*' refers to an ordinary everyday life. Japanese life in this analysis has a very close relationship with shrines. '*Hare*' refers to the time and space in which extraordinary events take place, including shrine festivals, annual events such as New Year's and seasonal festivals, and life rituals such as first shrine visits, *Shichigosan* (seven-five-three) and weddings and funerals (Miyata 2019:47–58). He clarified the difference between the two and said that Japanese life and culture can be analysed in terms of the cyclical rhythm of *hare* and *ke*.

On the day of *hare*, people change and put an end to the monotony of their daily lives, and on this day, people change their clothing, food and housing. Foods not eaten in daily life were offered to the guests, creating an extraordinary world. Yanagita notes that the purpose of drinking in the *hare* (celebratory occasions) was not so much to enjoy the taste as to experience abnormal psychology through intoxication, and to deepen the sense of solidarity among the people who made up the community by getting drunk together as a group. On the other hand, the *ke* time-space refers to the everyday state of life itself: waking up in the morning, eating, working during the day and resting at night.

Examining the connection between shrines and society in terms of *hare* and *ke* activities at shrines has developed around *hare*. The base of contact between shrines and people is the time and space where extraordinary events are held. Especially in Japan, where the population has been increasing since the post-war period, the increase in the birth rate has led to the mainstreaming of life rituals such as the first shrine visit, *Shichigosan*, and wedding ceremonies, which are important milestones in life, at shrines.

Festivals held at various shrines also symbolize the *hare* culture. The most important purpose of ceremonies is to please and entertain the *kami* by offering food (rice and other seasonal crops) and reciting words of thanksgiving and prayer. It is also a special day when the people of the community gather together to share their joy with *kami*. This is the scene of a lively ceremony. The community has deepened its unity by carrying the *mikoshi* (portable shrine) that the deity rides around the community during the festival, on their shoulders, skin to skin and by drinking and eating together at the end of the festival. Festivals have generated power through the so-called three-density state.

The limit of *hare* culture

The extraordinary time and space of the *hare*, which is created by such a dense concentration of people, is being lost, spurred by Covid. In other words, life rituals such as weddings and festivals and other opportunities for people to gather are being lost in the Corona disaster, where social distance is required. And the loss of the *hare* culture born of this density is actually showing signs even before Covid. Shrines, of which there are about 80,000 throughout Japan, have socially served as the centre of local communities. Shrines are still referred to as *Ujigami* (guardian *kami* of the local community) because of their long history of protection and transmission, supported by the reverence of the people who live in the community. However, the era of rapid population growth in Japanese society has come to an end, and the number of festival leaders and life rituals has been decreasing due to depopulation, the shift to nuclear families and a shrinking population. Due to this social trend, according to the research of Ishii Kenji, 41 per cent of all shrines in Japan may disappear by 2040. In other words, spurred by Covid, the existing model of running shrines through an extraordinary culture centred on prayers and festivals of life rituals has reached its limits.

As described above, the continuation of the existing shrine model, which focuses on *hare* culture, has become even more difficult, spurred by Covid. In order to break away from this existing shrine model, we predict that the future of shrines will require a 'theology of one shrine' and a 'culture of *ke*'. With the loss of the *hare* due to the Covid, an everyday culture symmetrical with the extraordinary, or the culture of *ke*, will be needed. In addition to special occasions such as life rituals and festivals, *ke* culture can be fostered by creating opportunities for people to visit shrines in their daily lives. In addition, when creating a culture of daily life, there is a need to build relationships with people outside the community, not limited to the local region, as the population decline and depopulation are accelerating in Japanese society. Therefore, the 'theology of one shrine' presented by Kenichi Shibukawa is helpful as a method for building connections outside the local region.

Each Shinto shrine must establish its own theology and then lead its own theology follower. Therefore, based on the divine virtues of the *kami* they serve, Shinto priests must form a single shrine, and at the same time, while speculating about the thoughts of the *kami* they serve, they must lead people under different conditions (Shibukawa 2008:133).

In Shinto, the world is thought to be made up of the workings of eight million *kami*. Each shrine has its own history and culture related to the *kami* it enshrines and has a unique story to tell. We argue that it is important for each shrine to design and tell a story from its history based on the blessings of its *kami*. It can be said that by assembling the theology of a single shrine, it is possible to create a living connection not only with the shrine's local community but also with people outside of that community.

The theology of one shrine and *ke* culture at Hattori Tenjingu Shrine

Based on the story of this theology of one shrine, Hattori Tenjingu Shrine in Osaka Prefecture is fostering everyday culture from the shrine side. Hattori Tenjingu is a shrine dedicated to the *kami* of feet, and in order to pass on the blessing of the *kami* of feet to people today, the shrine has launched an initiative to build daily culture for runners. With the increase in health awareness and Corona, the running population has been growing, and more and more people are visiting the shrine for running. Runners who wish for physical and mental health visit the Hattori Tenjingu Shrine to receive blessings from the *kami* of feet. The feet are the most important part of the body for running, and it is natural that people visit the *kami* of feet to pray for their health. In fact, running is an easy practice to implement in Corona as it avoids density, which is also the reason why it was adopted as a daily practice of the shrine. Therefore, we have launched a new initiative to create a daily culture of *ke* for runners. 'The Shrine Night Running', a project in which runners gather on the shrine grounds after the shrine gates are closed to pray at the shrine and then run in the neighbourhood, has been launched. The special feeling of being able to visit the shrine at night after the gates have closed has led to the creation of human connections around the shrine. The addition of praying to the *kami* of the feet to the daily rhythm of running helps foster physical and mental health. Furthermore, while the sense of loneliness has been intensified by Corona, the experience of being connected to people and nature through running has helped to solve the problem of loneliness. This is a case of everyday culture (*ke* culture) being nurtured based on one's own theology, the *kami* of feet, despite the Corona disaster.

The Corona has transformed the state of society, and even shrines that have maintained the status quo under the name of 'tradition' are now at a major turning point where change is required in order to survive. In the future, social conditions will continue to change drastically due to natural disasters and international situations of all kinds. We must be ready to change the direction of the inequality between *hare* and *ke* according to the changing times in the future. Rather than being biased towards one or the other, we should always form a culture that balances both *hare* and *ke*. It is important to prepare for the extraordinary while maintaining the everyday as the base and to be ready to revitalize the shrine through the return of these two aspects.

References

Hardacre, Helen. (2017). *Shinto: A History*. New York: Oxford University Press.

Ishii, Kenji. (2015). *Jinja Shinto to genkaishuraku* [Community Marginalization and Jinja Shinto]. Tokyo: Journal of Shinto Studies (237).

Miyata, Noboru. (2019). *Minzokugaku* [Folklore]. Tokyo: Kodansha.

Shibukawa, Kenichi. (2008). *Shouronshu* [Collections of Essay]. Tokyo: Jinja Shinpousha.

Yanagita, Kunio. (1969). *Yanagita Kunio zenshu daijyukan niihon no Matsuri* [Kunio Yanagita Collection Vol. 10 'Japanese Festivals']. Tokyo: Chikuma Shobo.

13

The significance of *matsuri* festivals in Shinto during epidemics

Koji Suga

The Japanese term 'Shinto' consists of two Chinese characters, *shin* (*kami*, deity, god) and *to* (way), as a whole meaning 'the way of *kami*'. Shinto is a polytheistic religion that emphasizes purification in its rituals for revitalization by enjoying the blessing and spiritual protection of *kami*. Shinto's practices are mainly based on performance of *matsuri* (rituals, ceremonies, festivals) in and around *jinja* (Shinto shrines).

In today's Japanese the word *matsuri* means festivals or lively events in general, whether religious or not. However, originally it is a noun form of the verb *matsuru*, which means to serve *kami*, to conduct rituals for worshipping *kami*. It is believed that these services and rituals should be related to communal interest rather than to an individual's desire. *Matsurigoto,* which is another noun form of this verb, is a classic expression of governance or politics. This shows that in ancient Japan religious rituals and political measures were undifferentiated as in other countries.

While Shinto originated in Japan, it is a country also known for its large Buddhist population. Presently there are almost eighty thousand Shinto shrines and several thousand fewer Buddhist temples in Japan. Most of these Shinto shrines and Buddhist temples today have no direct connections with each other in terms of religious practices and management. Regarding Japanese religious history, present Shinto's disconnection with Buddhism is a modern feature dating from 1868. At the time of the Meiji Restoration, the start of Japan's Western-style nation-state building, the new government proclaimed the separation of Buddhism from Shinto, against the amalgamation of these two which had been maintained more than one thousand years previously.

This Meiji new government was established under the banner of restoration of the imperial authority, calling for the revival of the mythological divine event of the first emperor's national foundation. While the authority of the imperial lineage as descendants of the sun goddess Amaterasu according to mythology has been respected throughout Japanese history, it came to be an important political issue in the middle of the eighteenth century as a feature of national identity in the face of Western colonialism in East Asia.

The officials of the early Meiji government intended to restore Shinto's original situation as it was in ancient times before the introduction of foreign Buddhism. Since then, along with the path of Japan's modernization, Shinto has reached its present form through a process of trial and error having its autonomy and its character as indigenous culture. After the failure of the state campaign to promulgate Shinto in the early Meiji period, state management of Shinto shrines as secular monuments for national history had been maintained for almost sixty years. Although the religious nature of Shinto shrines gradually gained attention in the latter part of these years, eventually it resulted in regarding shrines as local symbols for mobilizing people to total war. After Japan's defeat in the Second World War, Shinto shrines changed their legal status from 'non-religion' to 'religion' under the occupation by the Allied powers, and they remain so to this day under the principle of separation of state and religion.

Kami as the Object to Worship

Some scholars therefore assert that despite Shintoists' romanticized insistence on Shinto as timeless, unique spiritual culture based on customs rooted deeply in ancient Japan, most practices recognized as Shinto today are just a type of invented tradition for modern nationalism. Other scholars reject any dichotomy that differentiates 'indigenous' Shinto from other 'foreign' religions like Buddhism, Confucianism and Daoism since, as Helen Hardacre rightly points out, *kami* worship has absorbed much from these traditions (Hardacre 2107: 2-5). While considering their scepticism about the independence or uniqueness of Shinto, as a student of Shinto studies and a Shinto priest, I believe the question of how Shinto has reacted to the Covid-19 pandemic is worth answering as a case of religion's role in secularized society.

The word *kami* has been popular in Japanese vocabulary since ancient times though the term 'Shinto' in ancient documents meant not religious practices in a particular manner but matters about *kami* generally differentiated from Buddhism. As the other Shinto contributor to this book, Taishi Kato, also mentions (Chapter 12), probably the most convincing definition of *kami* as a Japanese word was given by the classics scholar Motoori Norinaga as follows:

> Those beings which possess extraordinary and surpassing abilities, and which are awesome and worthy of reverence are called 'kami', no matter whether they are good or evil.

> (Motoori [1790] 1968:53)

This definition of *kami* is still appropriate in today's Japanese vocabulary while additional elements mainly derived from the monotheistic concept of God as Christian divinity, like omnipotence, universal creator and saviour, have been included in some contexts. The important fact here is that Motoori reached this definition as a result of his detailed examinations of many mythological texts edited in the early eighth century and the classics after that time. This means that even the modern people who speak Japanese can understand the ancient relationship between *kami* and human beings. Interpreting Shinto generally as a human being's relationship towards *kami* – awe-inspiring spiritual beings with extraordinary and surpassing abilities – enables followers of those faiths to recognize Shinto as having been passed down from ancient times to the present day.

Matsuri and epidemics

Rituals to overcome epidemics must be one of the popular topics in Shinto history. The early examples can be seen even in the mythical-historical episodes of initial emperors. According to the *Nihongi* (Chronicle of Japan) edited in 720, during the rule of tenth emperor Sujin, a pestilence killed half of the population, and the civic situation became unstable. At that time, two *kami*, namely Amaterasu and Yamato-Ōkunitama were enshrined at the imperial residence. Because the emperor felt awe and was overwhelmed by having to cohabit with these two *kami*, he set up shrines to house these *kami* outside the imperial residence. Ancient records say that after moving around several locations, under the next emperor's reign, the precinct to enshrine Amaterasu was fixed permanently at where the Grand Shrine of Ise, the highest-ranked shrine, is today. The emperor Sujin also enshrined another kami Ōmononushi after divinations to overcome another plague, and this became the Ōmiwa shrine, one of the oldest shrines in Japan (Aston [1896] 1956:150–5, 176).

In general, in such ancient records, the causes of epidemics were understood as curses derived from deficiency of *matsuri* for worshipping particular *kami*. In other words, epidemics were interpreted as demands of some *kami* for sufficient worship. Later in the historical era in the eighth century, seasonal official Shinto rituals regulated in the legal code of the imperial court included several *matsuri* to prevent or quell epidemics.

Of course, under the modern principle of separating religion and state, the Japanese government in the twenty-first century never conducts any such official Shinto ritual to overcome the Covid-19 pandemic. In the recent situation, however, these examples in the ancient imperial court are usually cited as precedents of Shinto-style attempts to quell pandemics 1300 or more years ago. In today's situation, the ancient idea that the insufficiency of *matsuri* causes epidemics as a curse by *kami* must be reinterpreted in a secular way such as inadequate recognition of the menace being outside human scientific control causes misfortune.

The later historical cases of Shinto-Buddhist combined rituals to quell epidemics, whether civic or imperial, are also recognized as precedents for Japanese rituals to quell epidemics. The modern distinction between Shinto and Buddhism becomes a less serious matter in this context for Japanese tradition. Shinto shrines and Buddhist temples now respectively interpret such 'tradition' in their own distinctive ways, and apply such interpretations in their rituals, prayers, worships, distribution of amulets, and so on. Even some supernatural characters seen in early-modern folktales like *Amabie* or *Amabiko* become popular as 'traditional' charms. They are odd merman-like creatures with beaks who predicted either an abundant harvest or an epidemic and instructed people to make copies of their image to defend against illness. Today, Shinto shrines and Buddhist temples also join this fashion to distribute *Amabie*'s image together with sculptures, cartoon, and other illustrations (Shiromi 2020).

How has Covid-19 affected Shinto practices?

How has Covid-19 affected Shinto's religious practices, particularly in terms of the performance of *matsuri*? To see this point, we shall consider the Gion *matsuri* festival. While there are many Shinto rituals bearing the name Gion (this word has its origin in Buddhism) throughout Japan, the most famous one among them and the original is held at Yasaka shrine (classically called the Gion shrine) in Kyoto. To placate spirits of evil *kami* and revengeful dead who were thought to cause diseases and natural disasters, a Shinto-Buddhist combined style *matsuri* took place in Kyoto at the imperial court in 863. The expansion of such ritual to quell pestilences in 869 was regarded as the first Gion *matsuri* until today. This Gion *matsuri* includes the ceremonies outside the shrine, and the gorgeous procession of decorated floats as portable shrines going along the avenues in Kyoto city. This luxurious pageant at the capitol seems to have attracted large audiences, and it became the origin of spreading *matsuri* not only for worshipping *kami* but as festivals with pageants open to public view throughout the nation.

After the Covid-19 outbreaks, to prevent the spread of diseases the Japanese government has been urging people to avoid the 3Cs: 'Closed spaces with poor ventilation', 'Crowded places with many people nearby' and 'Close-contact settings such as close-range conversations'. To observe these requirements at least during the state of emergency declared, most events with a concentrated crowd in one place were suspended. The procession of floats of the Gion *matsuri* was also cancelled in July 2020 and July 2021.

Such cancellations of spectacular public events in *matsuri* were the typical responses of Shinto shrines and Buddhist temples to the government's statement to avoid 3C in ritual worship. Many other crowded ceremonies within shrines' *matsuri* throughout Japan, such as processions, collective prayers, dances and other votive performances, and communal feasts were abandoned. Most people understood the instruction, 'These *matsuri* are cancelled'. As I mentioned earlier, in today's common language the word *matsuri* is understood as a vibrant event. However, this is no longer quite accurate, because even at such events the core rituals of *matsuri* to worship *kami* were held by priests with limited attendances. Therefore, properly speaking, many *matsuri* as ritual worshipping of *kami* at shrines were held on a reduced scale during this emergency.

What we should reconsider

These responses to *matsuri* by the shrines to Covid-19 were based on observance of a series of notices by the Association of Shinto Shrines, the religious administrative organization that oversees about 97 per cent of all shrines throughout Japan. Here is an extract from this Association's notices, which was issued on 28 February 2020, shortly before the declaration of a state of emergency by the Japanese government:

Rituals should be performed. However, if the environment is such that the participants have to spend a certain amount of time indoors or in other places where there is not enough distance between them, which is considered a high risk of infection, the accompanying events like a communal feast and votive performances should be canceled or scaled back. And for events that gather an unspecified number of people, such as lectures held at shrines, consideration should be given to changing the timing of the event. In addition, when holding such events, specific measures to prevent infection (for example, washing hands, wearing masks, and so on) and thorough hygiene control of the building and shrine grounds should be taken, as necessary.

(Miyazawa 2022: 58–9)

Most of this statement is very similar to notices for holding secular events. Remarkably the first sentence 'Rituals should be performed' is the only content concerning religious faith mentioned here. This simple directive, which might even have been given by a former government official who was charged with the shrine's non-religious administration, was very important in this situation.

Although the original purpose of the Gion *matsuri* is to pray for quelling pestilence, and there are many traditional *matsuri* to pray for controlling the power of nature for human being society, as far as I know, no Shintoist professes scepticism about the protection of *kami* because such *matsuri* itself is forced to reduce its scale on account of pestilence. Also, there are no Shinto fundamentalists in general who argue that the rituals should never be changed to overcome the pestilence by the exorcism of *matsuri*.

Shinto may have become lost in the secular world behind the word 'tradition' in the history of modernization. Whether this is appropriate for a religion is an issue that should be considered as a consequence of the recent outbreak. Here we ought to consider another notice issued by the Association of Shinto Shrines on 1 July 2010, a decade earlier than the Covid-19 outbreak. This was a notice stating that so-called 'virtual worship' through shrines' websites must not be permitted because of the religious principles about Shinto shrines: 'The worship of Shinto shrines is based on the premise that one pays homage to a shrine where *kami* are enshrined and rituals are performed.' 'In principle, prayers must be made in person at the shrine' (Miyazawa 2022: 70).

As a theological reflection on this matter, I believe that the tension between human beings and awe-inspiring beings beyond human control, *kami*, in mediating between them, is what defines the sacred essence of *matsuri* religiously, even in the secularized society. This tension in the field of *matsuri* could never be replaced by today's advances in communication technology.

So, even after the Covid-19 pandemic is over, the religious emphasis on this tension must continue unabated in Shinto. *Matsuri* is a field of the interrelationship between human beings and *kami*. I believe that it will continue to have significance in today's highly secularized society as an expression of the coexistence between human beings and unknowable entities.

References

Aston, W. G. (trans.) ([1896]1956). *Nihongi*. London: George Allen & Unwin.

Hardacre, H. (2017). *Shinto: A History*. New York: Oxford University Press.

Miyazawa, Y. (2022). 'koronakaniokeru Jinjano taiouto kadai' in *Bulletin of C.P.E.R.E. 16*, 55–86, Kokugakuin University.

Motoori, N. ([1790]1968). *Kojikiden*, vol.1–11. Tokyo: Chikuma Shobo.

Shiromi, H. (2020). 'Plague-Fighting Monster Becomes Superstar as Pandemic Drags', *Asahi Shimbun*, 28 May. Accessible online at URL: https://www.asahi.com/ajw/articles/13370007.

Suga, K. (2018). 'Shinto'. In G. Oppy and N. Trakakis, eds., *Interreligious Philosophical Dialogues* vol.2. New York: Routledge.

14

Covid and *sewa*: Practising Sikhi during a global pandemic

Tejpaul Singh Bainiwal

Within a few months, the entire world came to a complete standstill with the Covid-19 pandemic. Schools, businesses and places of worship had all begun enforcing lockdown procedures to limit the spread of the virus. While the former two were able to eventually shift to a digital platform by allowing students and employees to attend school and work from home, emphasis was not placed on digital spaces for religious practices throughout Covid within the Sikh faith. Sikhs have been utilizing digital spaces pre-Covid; however, the pandemic was an opportunity to practise concepts that are central to the Sikh faith, such as *sewa* (selfless service), *nimarta* (humility) and *sarbat da bhala* (welfare of all). This chapter will explore how Sikhs applied these concepts to simultaneously (1) practise their faith during a global pandemic, (2) serve humanity and (3) educate individuals about the Sikh faith.

The spread of Covid

Sochai soch na hovaee je sochee lakh vaar
By thinking, God cannot be reduced to thought,
even by thinking hundreds of thousands of times.
Hukam rajae chalana nanak likhia naal
O Nanak, it is written that you shall obey the Hukam [Divine Order]
and walk in the way of God's Will.

Guru Nanak, *Jap Ji Sahib, Sri Guru Granth Sahib, 1*

In this opening prayer of the Guru Granth Sahib (Sikh scripture), Guru Nanak, the founder of the Sikh faith, writes *hukam rajae chalana nanak likhia naal.* While we struggle to understand why certain events occur – whether it be an oppressive government or a global pandemic, the Sikh faith teaches that everything happens according to *hukam* (Divine Order). We may never be able to truly understand why these events occur because it is beyond our thinking and cannot be reduced to thought. According to the Sikh faith, though we are unable to control these events, we can control our self. The Guru asks his Sikhs to 'practice truth, contentment, dharma, Name, charity, and ablution' (Bhai Gurdas Ji Vaar 11). Rather than attempting to explain Covid and dissect *hukam*, Sikhi focuses more on an internal journey and allowing one to follow Guru Nanak's message of 'cultivat[ing] true humility and be[ing] of service to others' (Grewal 1969: 185). Sikhi is a faith of action. The term, Sikh, itself means student and *sikhna,* which shares the same root word, means 'to learn'. Therefore, by accepting *hukam*, Sikhs can spend their time doing *sewa*, or selfless service through humility, which is one of the key tenets of the Sikh faith.

The tradition of *sewa* has been practised by Sikhs for over 500 years beginning with Guru Nanak. A well-known story within the Sikh tradition which highlights this practice is when Guru Nanak spent twenty rupees given to him by his father to start a business; instead Guru Nanak used the money to provide meals for a group of needy people. Guru Nanak's successor, Guru Angad, institutionalized a similar practice in the form of *langar* or community kitchen. The 500-year-old practice brings people from different caste, gender, religion, economic status and ethnicity together to share a simple vegetarian meal and ensure that hunger would never be a problem for anyone.

Another key institution for Sikhs is the *gurdwara*. Although some may define gurdwara to be solely a Sikh place of worship, there should be a heavy emphasis on the role it has played over the centuries and even today. Recognizing the gurdwara as simply a religious space strips away the importance of gurdwaras as sites for mobilizing the Sikh community for social, political and cultural causes. For example, Sikhs in Stockton, California, have been utilizing the gurdwara to mobilize for over a century. In 1915, the Stockton Gurdwara leadership stated that 'if a man is hungry and out of funds, we feed him. Our dining room is open at all hours of the day and is closed only for a few hours during the night. The unfortunate hungry American will be as welcome as our own people' ("Sikh Temple is Dedicated" 1915). For centuries, gurdwaras remained open despite ongoing wars or plagues as they adapted to the needs of the community. This pandemic proved to be the same. Religious services were temporarily stopped to abide by lockdown procedures while the importance of langar was elevated. Gurdwaras shifted their focus to adapt to the needs of the community by feeding millions of people worldwide during this global pandemic. The combination of *sewa* and *langar* has been the motivating factor behind serving those in need during the global pandemic, with gurdwaras oftentimes being the institution used to highlight these practices.

Sewa at Stockton, California

With concerns surrounding the pandemic, the Sikh community filled a void that many individuals were facing. As states began issuing mandatory statewide stay-at-home orders, many Sikhs refused. The reason? To provide groceries and essential items to those confined in their homes. Beginning mid-March 2020, several Sikh organizations and gurdwaras across the globe began to mobilize. Action is the heart of Sikhi and religious services are meant to help guide us to a path of *nimarta*, *sewa* and *sarbat da bhalla*. *Sewa* is a way of life and a part of daily routine. As Covid-19 spread, so did *sewa*. Sikhs stepped into lead roles where governments failed. They took the initiative to help as many people as possible who were affected by the drastic changes brought about by the pandemic (Bainiwal 2020). Although the lockdown banned or limited religious gatherings, gurdwaras across the globe stayed open to serve millions of people. To tell this global story, however, we can concentrate on efforts in San Joaquin County, California, United States.

In the heart of San Joaquin County sits Stockton Gurdwara, the first gurdwara in the United States. In April 2020, Stockton Gurdwara was set to commemorate the first initiation ceremony within the Sikh faith, *Khalsa Sajna Divas* or more commonly referred to as *Vaisakhi*. In 1699, Guru Gobind Singh (tenth Sikh Guru) initiated the first *Panj Piare* ('Cherished Five') to form the new Khalsa order. What would have been the twenty-first annual *Vaisakhi Nagar Kirtan*, a procession throughout the city celebrating the birth of the Khalsa, was halted due to the pandemic. However, rather than tens of thousands of Sikhs congregating at Stockton Gurdwara as happened in previous years, a group of Sikh youth met to set up the Sikh Pantry, a charitable organization started during the early months of the pandemic. Motivated by *sewa*, the Sikh Pantry delivered groceries and essential items during the lockdown to those in the greater San Joaquin County and the City of Modesto. Within the first three weeks, the Sikh Pantry was able to establish an online ordering system and deliver groceries and essential items to nearly five hundred families. Local elected officials even participated in the 'Sikh Pantry Drive Thru' event hosted at Stockton Gurdwara and assisted in helping the Sikh Pantry secure a grant to continue serving the community. Local Sikh-owned businesses donated dozens of pizzas (Mountain Mike's Pizza) and cupcakes (Kaur Cakery) for the

Sikh Pantry to deliver to frontline workers. Eventually, the Sikh Pantry was awarded the 'Key to the City' for their selfless service to the community. While practising their faith through serving others, the Sikh Pantry was also educating the local community about the Sikh faith and motivating more individuals to lend a hand, including many non-Sikhs.

Beyond groceries and essential items, a shortage of masks encouraged Sikhs to also distribute masks for those in need. Sikhs in Manteca (roughly twenty kilometres south of Stockton) initiated an effort to provide face masks for United States Postal Service workers. While an emphasis was placed on healthcare professionals and law enforcement officers as essential workers, Sikhs felt it was imperative for postal workers to be included in that category as they deliver important mail and many other essential documents to the community. Upon realizing that many workers and families were in need of masks, Sikhs across the county launched a full-fledged mask-sewing campaign. Local Sikh-owned small businesses donated cotton fabric, and Sikhs, primarily Sikh women, began sewing together masks from the comfort of their own home. Teams of Sikhs were tasked with supplying fabric to *sewadars* (those who are doing *sewa*) and picking them up when they are done. Masks were then delivered to anyone in need. Occasionally, Sikhs were able to secure N-95 masks, which were distributed to healthcare professionals and law enforcement officers during 'Mask and Hand Sanitizer Drives' at Stockton Gurdwara.

As the lockdown continued, so did the *sewa*. In Tracy, roughly twenty miles southwest of Stockton, and Lodi, ten miles north of Stockton, Sikhs turned their gurdwaras into Covid clinics. First, the gurdwaras offered drive-through Covid testing open for the public in which hundreds of tests were conducted at the peak of Covid. Shortly after, once vaccines became more available, gurdwaras across the county began offering Covid vaccinations. Within several months, the efforts at gurdwaras in Tracy, Lodi and Manteca resulted in the vaccination of over 50,000 individuals. Another area in which Sikhs have been in the frontlines is providing fresh meals to truck drivers. Truck drivers became some of the most essential workers across the nation to ensure groceries and other essential items are reaching communities. With over 100,000 Sikh American truck drivers across the United States, Sikhs understood the importance of truck drivers. Once they saw the hardships certain truck drivers were facing, Sikhs began serving free fresh meals to truck drivers outside a Safeway and Costco distribution centre in Tracy and at the Oakland Port. Beginning in Tracy, the group, standing on the side of the road, distributed hundreds of to-go meals. Over the next three meal distribution events (two in Tracy and one in Oakland), Sikhs distributed nearly 1,500 meals – 900 in Tracy and 550 in Oakland.

Practising sewa: The worldwide situation

The rapid spread of Covid left communities, of all backgrounds, stunned and the repercussions hit families in waves as different variants arrived. The story of Stockton, and its neighbouring cities, is merely a microcosm of what Sikhs have done throughout the world – some initiatives which were highlighted in the media and some not – to ensure they are making the world a better place despite the global pandemic. Sikhs put their personal health, and their family's health, on the line and risked themselves to exposure in order to ensure first responders, essential workers, senior citizens and everyone else were safe. Despite religious practices within gurdwaras being restricted, the pandemic was an opportunity for Sikhs to continue their religious practices and serve the community. *Sewa* throughout the Covid pandemic is interconnected with a longer history of service to the broader community as the concepts of *sewa* and *langar* have moved beyond the borders of gurdwaras. The call to serve, which is a core value of the Sikh faith, is only amplified in times of need as seen throughout the pandemic.

Throughout the Covid pandemic, Sikhs strongly felt that they should continue to serve those in need – especially since the need had grown to unexpected numbers. Food bank visitors grew by large percentages and the sudden change in lifestyle created a shortage of food and sanitary essentials. Sikhs rallied to serve the community the best they can and through whatever resources were available to them. Because of the already-established *langar*, at every gurdwara, Sikhs were able to provide large amounts of food in short periods of time. There was an influx of young Sikhs willing to buy and deliver groceries for those who were unable to leave their homes. Primarily Sikh women sewed together cloth face masks for frontline workers, including healthcare professionals, and helping those who may not (or did not) have access to masks such as low-income families and senior citizens. In addition to making masks, gurdwaras adapted to the needs of the community as they have done so in the past. Throughout the pandemic, any drastic change in religious practice was not necessary since service to the community through *sewa* and *langar* is a form of religious practice within the Sikh faith. It is a continuation of Guru Nanak's message of *sewa*. As mentioned earlier, the Sikh faith is centred around service and learning. So, while gurdwaras became a major source of food for millions of people worldwide during this global pandemic as Sikhs practised their faith, the next step is to learn how to become a better resource for the broader community. For example, Stockton Gurdwara is currently in the process of establishing a permanent health clinic and discussing the possibility of a permanent food bank. As society attempts to adjust to the new norm in a post-Covid world, Sikhs are considering how to ensure the long-term sustainability of *sewa* for the welfare of all. While accepting the pandemic to be within *hukam*, Sikhs focused more on how to practise their faith, through *sewa*, during a global pandemic.

References

Bainiwal, T. (2020). 'Sikhi, Seva, and Sarbat da bhalla in a Pandemic.' In D. Kenley ed., *Teaching about Asia in a Time of Pandemic*. Association for Asian Studies, 23–9.

Bhai Gurdas Ji, Accessible online at URL: www.sikhitothemax.org/.

Grewal, J. (1969). *Guru Nanak in History*. Chandigarh: Punjab University.

'Sikh Temple Is Dedicated'. *Stockton Record*. 22 November 1915.

15

Sikh scriptemics during pandemic

Nikky-Guninder Kaur Singh

> *dukh daru sukh rogu bhaia*
> Suffering is medicine; pleasure, the disease.
>
> (*GURU GRANTH SAHIB* [GGS]: 469)

How could suffering (*dukh*) be medicinal? With the onset of Covid-19, this paradoxical statement by Guru Nanak (1469–1539), the founder of the Sikh religion, began to make enormous sense. The unknown virus struck somewhere, and suddenly life across the globe was upended. Millions were dying lonely deaths, children were orphaned, pregnant mothers dying before they could make it to a hospital – everything taken for granted came to a standstill. Midst pain, fear, chaos, confusion, darkness and lockdown, Guru Nanak's positive take on suffering began to unfold. Indeed Guru Nanak's medicinal *dukkha* is an awakening from the stupor of daily dead habits. Tucked in our comfort zones with no deep reflection and drowned in daily pleasures (*sukha*), life is lived narrowly and selfishly. Our collective *dukkha* suddenly made us cognizant of a larger reality. We begin to wonder what is really important. What is the meaning and purpose of life?

Reflecting on some key Nanakian values tends to have a medicinal efficacy. He celebrates human origins in the mother's womb, our body and senses, our biophilial existence, human unity and equality, our being together socially and environmentally, and working for the collective good. What he lyrically expressed was also reiterated by his successors and recorded in scripture, the Guru Granth Sahib (GGS), which I refer to as 'Sikh scriptemics'. This 1430-page text spanning several centuries and authors from diverse religious and social backgrounds, is a rich reservoir of the ideals, values, perceptions and imagination launched by Guru Nanak. At this agonizing hour, its joyous and inclusive notes are profoundly effective. In fact, they serve as an antidote to 'infodemic' which is polarizing global society. As the World Health Organization has stated, 'infodemic' is inaccurate and false information circulating about the pandemic – how the virus originated, its cause, its treatment and its mechanism of spread – that has increased hate speech and human rights violations (WHO 23 September 2020). In contrast, the transcendent Sikh scriptemic melodies, intersecting with our Covid-stricken temporality, bring much solace; they provide a critical diagnosis of our current human behaviour, and they inspire us to take action for the future.

Preciousness of birth and biophilial existentiality

'This birth is precious as a diamond – *hire jaisa janam hai*' (GGS:156) is the *leitmotif* of Guru Nanak's poetics. In contrast with 'necrophilic imaginary' of patriarchal theology which feminist philosophers have been warning against (Cavarero 1995:69), Guru Nanak shifts the focus from death and afterlife to our very origins in this world. Life and living in diverse forms are fully affirmed: 'Born from egg, womb, sweat, or earth, Your light pulsates in every heart' (GGS: 1109).

In a melody of phonetic sounds and a collage of visual images, Guru Nanak photographs the spiritual textures in the creative site of pregnancy:

Semen and blood came together to create the body;
Air, water, fire came together to create life;
And the One performs wonders in the colorful body;
all else is the expanse of illusion and attachment.
In the rounded womb is the upside-down thinker,
And the knower knows every one's hearts;
Each breath remembers the true name,
for inside the womb flourishes the One.

(GGS: 1026–7)

This is no scopophilic or fetishistic construction. Casting light on the maternal organ, the Guru takes his audience back to that magical location where life is produced – life that is the body, life that is the spirit. Physical elements – air (*paun*) water (*pani*) fire (*agni*) – combine to produce the foetus fondled lovingly by the universal Divine. Turned upside down, the foetus remembers (*samale*) the true (*sac*) name (*nam*) with each and every breath (*sas sas*), while feeding on the nutrients of the physical elements which the mother herself shares with the rest of the cosmos. Spiritual incubation in the intrauterine phase is a vital ontological scene.

Coming into the world, our basic act of breathing palpitates with biophilial existentiality. This world is real, for it is a part of Truth: 'air is produced by Truth and from air comes water' (GGS: 19). The epilogue of Nanak's Japji captures a warm holistic scenario:

> Air is our guru, water is our father
> The unifying womb, our mother earth
> Night and day are the two male and female nurses
> This is how You keep the play of the world playing.

That air is identified as the guru signifies that we humans have the same one teacher, and that our 'knowledge' comprises each breath informing us about the vast singular reality keeping the momentum of the creative play. Earth is the mother, the matrix from which we all originate, and father is water which is approximately 80 per cent of our bodies. Night and day are our male and female nurses who look after us. The verb 'playing' (*khelai*) intimates our delightful movements in the rhythmic lap of night and day – with the awareness of the infinite One each moment as we breathe (*air is our guru*). Life is always now. Being is in the present.

Unfortunately, puffed up with haughty air and engrossed in selfish I-me pursuits, we remain oblivious. Witnessing millions being ravaged by the respiratory syndrome reveals the criticality of the simple act we perform night and day, along with the vitality of the primal element 'air' we share with our fellow beings biotic and abiotic. Not eternity out there, but each and every minute of this ever-changing world is vital. Progress and science are a part of our historical reality. We must get vaccinated; we must wear masks – not merely for ourselves but for the protection of our fellow beings. With the minuscule ferocious virus constantly mutating, new discoveries and better healthcare are urgently needed. We cannot let politics or religion divide us.

Somatophilial orientation

The importance of the bodily senses, so powerfully exhibited by Covid, evokes a somatophilial orientation. But the body and its senses have been denounced by lovers of ideas and ideals like Plato along with body-denying ascetics from various religious traditions. The mind-body dualism seismic across cultures is dangerous for emotional health, and for the social, political, economic and environmental infrastructures. How can we think or exist without our bodily senses? Guru Nanak passionately addresses the infinite One 'to You belong my breath, to You my flesh; says poet Nanak, you are our true Provider' (GGS: 660). His distinctive way of conceiving and perceiving through the body was a new way of being with Being that he set into motion in medieval India, and it serves as a valuable model for our dualized selves in the polarized society we inhabit.

The senses of smell and taste have been particularly hit by Covid, and their devastating loss calls for a reassessment of Kant's dictum: 'To which organic sense do we owe the least and which seems to be the most dispensable? The sense of smell. It does not pay us to cultivate it or to refine it in order to gain enjoyment' (Kant 1978: 46). Smell is linked to emotion and memory, and its loss (anosmia) is associated with depression (Valencia 3 June 2021). Centuries ago Guru Nanak proclaimed the ability to smell essential for knowledge and spirituality: 'Only the person who enjoys the fragrance knows the flower' (GGS:725).

Likewise, Covid has showcased the significance of the sense of taste, which again is denigrated by mind-exalting intellectuals (Korsmeyer 1999). Sikh scriptemics invoke taste with great gusto through an embodied experience. The tongue drenched in the flavours of the infinite One is an immediate gustatory experience, and as a lingering aftertaste maintains temporal continuity with the present. In this sense taste is unique among the senses as the other four have no equivalent of aftertaste such as aftersight, or aftertouch, or aftersound, or aftersmell. Guru Nanak's topos has an ontological bite: The universal One is the primal cause and ultimate saviour: 'ape rasia ape rasa ape ravanhar – Itself the relisher, Itself the taste, it Itself is the bestower' (GGS: 23). Senses are a precious gift, and to be healthy, we must treasure them and continue to refine all five of them. For these, according to Guru Nanak, can develop into truth, contentment, compassion, righteousness and patience, or they can regress into lust, anger, greed, attachment and pride.

Unity across religions and social equality

Guru Nanak's foundational statements – there is only one reality (ikk oan kar) and that there is only one moral compass (eko dharam) for humans – replay across Sikh scriptemics. Both these are poignantly brought to light by the virus attacking everybody – Hindu, Muslim, Jew, Christian, Parsi or Bahá'í alike. It made no exceptions as it glided past religious borders that we humans unnecessarily construct and solidly uphold. And it attacked everyone irrespective of race, class or gender hierarchies. Covid-19 is a powerful reminder that we originate from the same matrix and have the same human responsibilities. Sadly, the facts go against. The pandemic has not only exposed but also augmented deep-rooted religious, racial, class and gendered inequalities. Unemployment, mental health, domestic violence, poverty have but increased.

The severe lockdown in India was horrendous for migrant labourers who lost their wages and some even their life from starvation or suicides as they were forced to trek back to their remote villages. 'The lockdown and social security measures were implemented in a "top-down manner" which resulted in acute economic distress of the urban poor,' observes Nadira Singh (2022: 2).

In the land where Guru Nanak championed oneness and equity of Hindus and Muslims, the latter have been stigmatized for super-spreading coronavirus. After a meeting of the Tablighi Jamaat, an Islamic group, hashtags such as 'CoronaJihad', 'CoronaTerrorism', 'Talibanicrime' and 'CoronaBombsTablighi' began to circulate. Because of the 'infodemic' Islamic conspiracy to spread the virus to Hindus nationwide, hundreds of Muslim houses and shops were vandalized.

In North America anti-Asian hate crimes and discrimination increased dramatically. In spite of their presence for over a century in Canada and the United States, Sikhs continue to remain the *Other*. Because of their items of faith, they are easily visible, and targeted. In the tragic shooting at a FedEx facility there were four Sikh Americans murdered by a white supremist (Indianapolis, 15 April 2021).

The uncut Sikh beards and hair (*kesha*) are a marker of the natural gift from the divine One. For Sikh frontline workers, paramedics, nurses, doctors, dentists and first responders, tight-fitting filtering facepiece (FFP3) face masks are essential respiratory protective equipment and require a fit test to assess mask–face seal competency. However, facial hair is an impediment for achieving a competent seal. Going through an existential crisis between precepts of faith and professional commitment, two Sikh doctors in Canada shaved their beards to treat Covid-19 patients (Elassar 16 May 2020). The Legal Director of the Sikh Coalition Amrith Kaur explains that observant Sikhs not given accommodations to facially neutral employment policies and regulations is a part of the systemic discrimination against minorities in the United States (Kaur 28 April 2021).

An insightful study unravels issues of race and media in the Canadian cities of Brampton and Alberta that have large Sikh populations. It highlights neo-racism, a phenomenon of culturalist racism which is 'not biological inferiority of the migrant non-national other' but a corrosion of Canada's multiculturalism (Gupta and Nagpal 2022: 103–22). Pivoting on cultural essentialism and incommensurability of pre-modern South Asian values, Canadian media attributed the high Covid cases amongst Sikh Punjabis to their multi-generational families and traditional lifestyles. There was no mention of White anti-masker rallies in the same cities nor of the socio-economic conditions of the Sikh Punjabis concentrated 'in precarious employment such as truck driving, warehouse, janitorial and cleaning work, which lack paid sick leaves, job security and living wages. In these occupations workers do not have the luxury of operating from their homes, observing social distance and staying home when they are starting to feel ill' (Gupta and Nagpal 2022: 110–11).

The process of recognizing the rupture between our essential unity and the dangerous divisions and polarizations we have succumbed to, we hope, should give us ammunition to make the world a better place for all of us.

Sewa

Sewa or selfless service is a pivotal institution begun by Guru Nanak. His basic exhortation 'Living in this world, let us serve – *vic dunia sev kamaia*' (GGS: 26) is reinforced by his successors. 'To serve is to shed the egoistic I-me'(GGS: 407); "when I serve, my mind suffuses in love (GGS: 490). World-affirming *sewa* sheds selfish ego, transcends individuality and, infusing love within, motivates dynamic action for 'the good of all – *sarbat da bhala*' (finale of Sikh prayer 'Ardas').

The pandemic saw Sikh men and women implementing *sewa* most innovatively, most energetically with 'body, mind, and wealth' (*tan man dhan*) as the saying goes. Across the globe they took up amazing humanitarian initiatives. The typical community meal (*langar*) cooked, served and partaken in gurdwaras broadened in many ways including 'take out' and 'delivery' services. Gurdwara Bangla Sahib in New Delhi, for instance, committed itself to 'Langar on Wheels' – daily fifteen vans dispatched to serve food to the hungry and destitute in 'Jhuggi-Jhopri clusters, railways stations, bus stands, rain shelters and pavements' (Agrawal 3 June 2020).

Diasporic Sikh communities across the globe have been supplying basmati rice, lentils, vegetable dishes to hospital workers, the homeless, the elderly or anyone in search of a hot meal. Even lorry drivers stuck in Kent due to UK–France travel ban had *langar*! Since Punjabi dishes are part of the *Other's* diet, Canadian media has been familiarizing mainstream audiences by using analogies like 'trick or treat' for their packaging, and emphasizing masks, gloves and hygienic methods in their preparation (Gupta and Nagpal 2022: 103–22). During oxygen shortage crisis, Sikh gurdwaras and NGOs opened life-saving medical 'Oxygen Langars', and converted some Langar halls into Covid care centres with oxygen beds.

A perfect example of *sewa* is Jatinder Singh Shunty – the embodiment of humanitarianism, heroism, pluralism and relentless service. At the peak of Covid, he took up the job of the untouchables to perform the last rites of Covid contagious patients. According to their respective traditions, Hindu, Muslim, Sikh and Christian dead were cremated or buried with dignity. Clearly Guru Nanak's ideals of the One reality, *ikk oan kar*, and one morality, *eko dharam*, are put into actual practice.

Overcoming the fear of death

The pandemic has escalated fear and anxiety. 'Why fear fear? We belong to the One, so what's there to fear?' reassures Guru Nanak (GGS: 796). In fear of tomorrow we lose the present. Guru Nanak squarely makes us confront death and helps overcome the much-feared phenomenon: 'Death would not have a bad name if only people knew what death is' (GGS: 579). The Guru's new and heroic impulse is greatly praised: 'Such language was unique in an age dominated by timidity and apprehensiveness. Death was not to be regarded as the unspeakable dread that crippled every moment of life, but the portal by which men entered a new realm of God's wisdom and love' (Singh 1969: 214). The Sikh approach to suffering and death is that of serene acceptance: 'may we taste the sweetness of Your will – mitha lagai tera bhana' (GGS: 543). There is no retribution. Like night and day, sukh-dukh constitute the fabric of life – a part of the ticking of time in the cosmic motion of lunar and solar systems making up seasons, dates, days, hours and seconds. The finale of Sikh funeral resounds 'jewel-like melodies with their families and fairies (parian) from afar have come to sing the holy word within' (Hymn of Bliss/ Anand). Death ceremony entails family and friends sitting in the presence of the GGS and listening to its uplifting melodies. During Covid restrictions, Zoom became the channel for such gatherings (sangat).

Conclusion

Keynote of Sikh scriptemics – the consanguineous relationship with the world at large – is strikingly brought home by Covid-19. Any tiny virus in any part of the world can impact any one of us and will affect all of us. We are all a part of the vast living, breathing, planetary organism. Such realization radically shifts the view of human dominion over nature in terms of partnership and kinship with nature, and a commitment to justice for all beings. We are forced to be self-critical: we humans are one species in the system, a part of nature, so how did we get to be the 'owners'? Is it not time we shake off our arrogance and dominance? Is it not time to put away our selfish motives and work for the good of all? What Guru Nanak characterized *dukkha* actually leads to healing and wholesomeness.

References

Agrawal, Palak. (3 June 2020). Delhi: For Poor Who Can't Find Nearest Gurudwara, Sikh Community Launches 'Langar on Wheels'. Accessible online at URL: https://thelogicalindian.com/app-lite/news/delhi-gurudwara-langar-on-wheels-feeds-needy-covid-19-21462.

Cavarero, Adriana. (1995). *In Spite of Plato*. New York: Routledge.

Elassar, Alaa (Saturday, 16 May 2020). CNN report. Accessible online at URL: https://edition.cnn.com/2020/05/16/health/sikh-doctors-beards-coronavirus-trnd/index.html.

Gupta, T. D. and S. Nagpal. (2022). 'Unravelling Discourses on COVID-19, South Asians and Punjabi Canadians' in *Studies in Social Justice* 16 (1). Accessible online at URL https://journals.library.brocku.ca/index.php/SSJ/article/view/3471.

Kant, Immanuel, (trans.) V. L. Dowdell. (1978). 'On the Five Senses'. In H. H. Rudnick. ed. *Anthropology from a Pragmatic Point of View*. Carbondale: Southern Illinois University Press: 40–48.

Kaur, Amrith. (28 April 2021). 'Written Testimony of Amrith Kaur, Legal Director, Sikh Coalition' US Equal Employment Opportunity Commission. Accessible online at URL: https://www.eeoc.gov/meetings/meeting-april-28-2021-workplace-civil-rights-implications-covid-19-pandemic/kaur.

Korsmeyer, Carolyn. (1999). *Making Sense of Taste*. Ithaca, NY: Cornell University Press.

Singh, Harbans. (1969). *Guru Nanak and Origins of the Sikh Faith*. Bombay: Asia Publishing House.

Singh, Nadira. (2022). 'Sikhism and Covid-19: Ethics of Community Service and Activism', *Sikh Formations: Religion, Culture, Theory*. Accessible online at URL: www.tandfonline.com/doi/full/10.1080/17448727.2022.2084946.

Valencia, David. (3 June 2021). Featured Topic: 'Covid-19 and Loss of Smell, Taste', Mayo Clinic.

World Health Organization. (23 September 2020). 'Managing the COVID-19 Infodemic: Promoting Healthy Behaviours and Mitigating the Harm from Misinformation and Disinformation'. Joint statement by WHO, UN, UNICEF, UNDP, UNESCO, UNAIDS, ITU, UN Global Pulse and IFRC.

All translations from the Sikh Scripture, the Guru Granth Sahib (GGS), are by the author.

16

Navigating the Covid-19 pandemic: Building resilience: Reflections of a Bahá'í

Wendi Momen

Encountering Covid

I had just arrived in New York for my annual participation in the UN Commission on the Status of Women (CSW) and was travelling from the airport when I learned that the United Nations was closing all its premises to everyone that very day for an unspecified time. The two-week CSW Summit was cancelled, and only the government members of the Commission would debate, remotely, the issues affecting all women in the year ahead. Aaargh!

CSW 2020 was supposed to celebrate the 25th anniversary of the 4th UN Conference on Women held in Beijing in 1995, which had established the Platform for Action, the bible for the advancement of women across the globe. I had been at that historic event and was now part of a team from the National Alliance of Women's Organisations (NAWO) in the UK that had brought twenty-six high school girls to speak at CSW side events. These were cancelled. Pretty much everything was closed. We could not change our flights home.

This was my introduction to Covid-19 as something more than just a very unpleasant flu-like illness. Here was one of the biggest cities in the world closing down. People were afraid, confused, angry and began to panic buy. Not knowing how to navigate this situation, the little NAWO team, four Bahá'ís and two others who had arrived in New York together, met in the hotel where the young women were staying. We had to do something to enable them to have a meaningful and fulfilling programme for a week, as even sightseeing was impossible. The young women had written short speeches on the CSW themes for that year: the current challenges affecting the implementation of the Platform for Action and the achievement of gender equality, and the empowerment of women and its contribution towards the realization of the 2030 Agenda for Sustainable Development.

Trying to remain calm and positive, and recalling the prayer that begins 'Be calm, be strong, be grateful' ('Abdu'l-Bahá 1915: 405), we invoked the Bahá'í concept of consultation to determine what to do: pray; identify the issue; ascertain the facts, incorporate expert or other information; identify the spiritual principles involved; put ideas forward; detach oneself from owning the idea; discuss all ideas to uncover the truth and determine the way forward; decide by consensus or majority agreement; support the decision, even if you do not agree with it; implement the decision.

We considered the health implications, which no one really understood, took the health advice available at the time and decided to ask the hotel for a room large enough for about 35 people. We created an ad hoc programme at which each woman could present her talk and hear speakers representing different governments, agencies and organizations. We called on local friends, our colleagues from Soroptimist International (a global women's organization), contacts from US agencies and our own and other governments to participate. We created an eight-day programme, with two or three guests attending each session. The Bahá'í friend I was staying with, a playwright whose off-Broadway show 'Sistas' played the day after we arrived and then closed for two years, pitched up to give talks about her work. Soroptimists came on a rota to listen to the speeches and give talks about women's empowerment. A UN representative answered questions, and UK diplomats explained what the government was doing to advance women. It was not what we had come for, but it worked.

Eventually able to get on the last but one plane to the UK before flights were restricted, I returned home to a different world with a new vocabulary – social distancing, PPE, Zoom, lockdown, shielding and, later, lateral flow tests, PCRs – and a whole new set of actions – washing hands while singing Happy Birthday, spraying doorknobs with bleach, wearing a mask and rubber gloves while shopping for essentials, spending hours and hours in front of my computer teaching, attending conferences and many many meetings each day. I also increased the amount of time I read Bahá'í scriptures each day and prayed for a growing list of family members and friends with Covid, for those who had passed away from Covid, those whose spouse, child or parent had Covid or had passed away, those whose wedding, hospital appointment, school or university classes had been cancelled – and meditated on the meaning of it all.

Trying to understand

So what *was* the meaning of it all? As a political scientist, one passage from the Bahá'í texts had always intrigued me. Shoghi Effendi, the great grandson of the founder of the Bahá'í Faith, Bahá'u'lláh, had written in his capacity as head and Guardian of the religion a lengthy letter in 1936 to the Bahá'ís of the West outlining Bahá'u'lláh's teachings on the 'Unfoldment of World Civilization'. In it he described the effect the universal recognition of the oneness of humanity would have on society, mentioning:

Destitution on the one hand, and gross accumulation of ownership on the other, will disappear. The enormous energy dissipated and wasted on war, whether economic or political, will be consecrated to such ends as will extend the range of human inventions and technical development, to the increase of the productivity of mankind, *to the extermination of disease, to the extension of scientific research, to the raising of the standard of physical health, to the sharpening and refinement of the human brain ... to the prolongation of human life,* and to the furtherance of any other agency that can stimulate the intellectual, the moral, and spiritual life of the entire human race.

(Shoghi Effendi 1991:204; author's italics)

So, here we were in a pandemic and one way to prevent further pandemics is to accept the reality that we are one people living on one planet, redirect our resources away from destruction and use them for these health and life-affirming purposes instead. This is not simple but it is possible, even inevitable. Reflecting on this and on what was happening, I saw that the global race to create vaccines was accelerated when governments and scientists cooperated. Health outcomes improved when people were put before profits, when knowledge was shared. We could do this.

This interplay of spiritual belief and its application in social reality is characteristic of the Bahá'í Faith and for the most part shaped the response of individual Bahá'ís, their communities and their institutions to the pandemic. Bahá'ís are called to:

Quench ye the fires of war, lift high the banners of peace, work for the oneness of humankind and remember that religion is the channel of love unto all peoples.

('Abdu'l-Bahá 1978: 35)

Taking action

That humanity has not yet accepted its oneness motivates Bahá'ís to increase their efforts to share the teachings of Bahá'u'lláh with others, especially well-wishers of humanity, and particularly this concept of the oneness of humanity, which is the foundation of all the Bahá'í social principles. At the same time, Bahá'ís are called to be of service to humanity at all times:

> Be ye the helpers of every victim of oppression, the patrons of the disadvantaged. Think ye at all times of rendering some service to every member of the human race. Pay ye no heed to aversion and rejection, to disdain, hostility, injustice: act ye in the opposite way. Be ye sincerely kind, not in appearance only. Let each one of God's loved ones centre his attention on this: to be the Lord's mercy to man; to be the Lord's grace. Let him do some good to every person whose path he crosseth, and be of some benefit to him.
>
> ('Abdu'l-Bahá 1978: 3)

So in ways large and small, Bahá'ís, like millions of others, found ways to be of some service to neighbours, friends and not-yet-friends. My New York playwright friend spent hours sewing hundreds of masks, giving away handfuls to passers-by. In our small community the Bahá'ís shopped for neighbours; cleaned their homes; helped children by providing art materials, books and online children's classes; served as marshals at test sites, said prayers with friends at their doors or on the phone; cooked meals for others; collected food for food banks; and paid weekly tribute to the National Health Service workers.

Junior youth, between 12 and 15, both Bahá'ís and others, helped those younger than themselves with reading and homework, organizing activities such as crafts, baking and physical exercises on Zoom to keep up spirits and foster friendships. People tried to forge meaningful friendships through Zoom conversations on themes of race, social justice and well-being; others created online friendship spaces in response to the loneliness, isolation and anxiety experienced by so many. Some responded to food shortages by delivering food packages and coordinating food banks. A community garden was created in one neighbourhood to provide fresh vegetables and a space where friends could gather safely outside, giving rise to conversations that resulted in projects such as book exchanges and winter coat collections. Bahá'ís working with newly arrived refugees created English-language programmes, literacy support and the use of the arts to help alleviate mental health issues.

These fledgling efforts by Bahá'ís and friends contributed a drop to the ocean of service provided by thousands and thousands of other well-wishers of humanity across the country.

Relying on divine guidance

As that timeless time went on, I began to realize how other Bahá'í principles inspired our conduct, for example, the need for individuals to search for the truth for themselves and the concept that 'science and religion are two complementary systems of knowledge and practice by which human beings come to understand the world around them and through which civilization advances' (Universal House of Justice 2013). These enabled individuals and families to decide whether or not to vaccinate when vaccines became available. Guidance coming from the Universal House of Justice, the international elected governing body of the Bahá'í world community, indicated that Bahá'ís needed to make such decisions themselves, based on consultation and the best expert advice they could identify. At the same time, it was pointed out that Bahá'ís also need to be conscious of the social implications of their decisions and their responsibility towards the community at large and the well-being of the whole of humanity.

The Bahá'í institutions also pointed out that we are living at a time when truth is sometimes hard to determine, as the media, especially social media, can so easily be used by people with certain agendas, masquerading as experts, to spread misinformation, rumours, conspiracy theories and falsehoods. It was suggested that Bahá'ís search for truth and understanding by trying to weed out sources that appear to be biased, unreliable or offering unsubstantiated views for partisan purposes, and to determine the consensus of reliable sources. This was not so easy but something Bahá'ís have always been encouraged to do.

Another teaching that enabled Bahá'ís to decide how to conduct themselves, particularly during lockdown and the period of limited social contact was 'each and every one is required to show obedience, submission and loyalty towards his own government' ('Abdu'l-Bahá 1978: 293), thus reminding the Bahá'ís to follow all government regulations and guidelines, whether or not others were obeying them.

Would praying help?

Like so many people around the world, during the pandemic I was praying for family, friends, health workers, all humanity. Did I think it would help? I did. The Bahá'í texts tell us that if we 'recite any of the revealed prayers, and seek assistance from God with thy face turned towards Him, and implore Him with devotion and fervour, thy need will be answered' ('Abdu'l-Bahá 2019). Further:

> The true worshipper, while praying, should endeavour not so much to ask God to fulfil his wishes and desires, but rather to adjust these and make

them conform to the Divine Will. Only through such an attitude can one derive that feeling of inner peace and contentment which the power of prayer alone can confer.

(Shoghi Effendi 1938)

Believing this, in addition to our usual daily prayers, my husband (who had to shield) and I started a weekly devotional meeting online on Saturday nights, beginning 4 April 2020 when the Bahá'ís launched a Day to Pray, an activity we have held every week since with people from different religions offering prayers in a short unscripted programme with music. This was the substitute for the monthly devotional meetings we began in our home in 2000 for neighbours. Another small action. We hope it is helpful.

But why a pandemic?

I still wanted to know why the pandemic happened? If God acts in the world, did He cause it to take place? Was it His will? If so, why? One statement of Bahá'u'lláh ran through my mind, heart and soul throughout those years, and still: 'Be generous in prosperity, and thankful in adversity' (Bahá'u'lláh 1983: 285). How to do this?

This brought me to the Bahá'í writings on resilience, tests and difficulties, and suffering. Bahá'ís do not consider tests and suffering to be punishments from God but part of human life:

Regarding your question about prayer and the fact that some of our problems are not solved through prayer, we must always realize that life brings to us many situations, some of which are tests sent from God to train our characters, some of which are accidental because we live in the world of nature and are subject to the accidents of death, disease, etc., and some of which we bring on ourselves by folly, selfishness or some other weak human trait.

(Shoghi Effendi 1951)

Some tests and difficulties may indeed be part of God's plan for us – a way to develop our character:

The mind and spirit of man advance when he is tried by suffering. The more the ground is ploughed the better the seed will grow, the better the harvest will be. Just as the plough furrows the earth deeply, purifying it of weeds and thistles, so suffering and tribulation free man from the petty affairs of this worldly life until he arrives at a state of complete detachment. His attitude in this world will be that of divine happiness. Man is, so to speak, unripe: the heat of the fire of suffering will mature him.

('Abdu'l-Bahá 1967: 178)

But what of collective suffering, I was wondering. This pandemic, for example, which has killed so many people, natural disasters or wars for which we as individuals are not responsible? Why do they happen? Why does God allow innocent people to suffer? So, as a result of my reflections I developed a distance learning course, currently running, with the Wilmette Institute in Chicago, to explore these questions with others, Bahá'í and non-Bahá'í. As I write there are twenty-eight of us from the UK, Malawi, China, the United States and Canada studying the Bahá'í texts and other scriptures, learning from each others' experiences, sharing insights. We are exploring this idea.

We can look at this issue (why God permits suffering) from the point of view of the source of the suffering. Much suffering in the world is brought on by ourselves, whether as individuals, groups of people or the whole world community. Wars, poverty, racism, abuse and injustices of all kinds are things we can actually get rid of but do not. Even some natural disasters seem to be caused, or exacerbated, by our neglect or abuse of the planet, while we consign some people to areas prone to such natural events and do not provide protection and aid when required. From the Bahá'í perspective, this is precisely why the great teachers from God (Abraham, Moses, Krishna, Zoroaster, Jesus, Buddha, Muhammad, Bahá'u'lláh) appeared – to enable humanity to follow the teachings of God and to correct the misdirections of their personal and collective lives. These great teachers have given us the tools and methods we need to better the world but many turn away from them.

We are still developing our thoughts about this. Learning, as we know, is a lifelong process. So in the end, I do not know whether the pandemic was sent by God to test humanity, or whether it was something we could have avoided by bending our energies to operationalizing God's guidance, or whether it was completely accidental. However, I have learned that it is one thing to read, to meditate and to become. It is another to do. Being and doing are two parts of our life's work. Thus has it been during Covid for this Bahá'í.

References

'Abdu'l-Bahá (1967). *Paris Talks*. London: Bahá'í Publishing Trust.
'Abdu'l-Bahá (2019). *Prayer and Devotion Life, a Compilation*. Haifa: Bahá'í World Centre.

'Abdu'l-Bahá (1915). *Tablets of Abdul-Baha Abbas*, vol. 2. Chicago: Bahá'í Publishing Society.

'Abdu'l-Bahá (1978). *Selections from the Writings of 'Abdu'l-Bahá*. Haifa: Bahá'í World Centre.

Bahá'u'lláh (1983). *Gleanings from the Writings of Bahá'u'lláh*. Wilmette, IL: Bahá'í Publishing Trust.

Shoghi Effendi (1938). From a letter written on behalf of Shoghi Effendi to an individual, 26 October.

Shoghi Effendi (1951). From a letter written on behalf of Shoghi Effendi to an individual, 18 March.

Shoghi Effendi (1991). *The World Order of Bahá'u'lláh*. Wilmette, IL: Bahá'í Publishing Trust.

The Universal House of Justice, Letter to the Bahá'ís of Iran, 2 March 2013.

17

World-embracing vision against world-threatening pandemic

George Merchant Ballentyne

I look on my pandemic experience as being in two equivalent parts, which unfolded alongside each other. One, outward-facing engagement with communities in Leicester, assisting in their response to and recovery from Covid-19; the other, inward-facing, behind closed doors, including two bouts of coronavirus and the necessary self-isolation, amid twenty months' working from home. I cannot separate one from the other. I hope this chapter will convey something of how my beliefs, principles and practices as a Bahá'í impacted both aspects.

Engagement with diverse local communities

Throughout this period, I was Voluntary and Community Sector Engagement Manager in the City Mayor's Office at Leicester City Council – a post I held for eight years in all (2013–21). For seven years before that (2006–13) I was Equality and Diversity Officer at Leicester Council of Faiths. When lockdown came in April 2020, I had under my belt fourteen years' professional engagement with groups, organizations and institutions identifying with the protected characteristics described in the Equality Act 2010. My acknowledged specialism was the protected characteristic of religion or belief, working with diverse faith and cultural communities.

Leicester endured lockdown for a longer continuous period than anywhere else in the UK. Covid-19 infection hotspots were located in city neighbourhoods associated with particular cultures, ethnicities and religions. Restrictions remained in force in Leicester long after they were eased elsewhere. The diversity that had been the jewel in Leicester's crown was decried by some as endangering the entire population.

The faith and cultural communities of Leicester took quite a pounding. Yet these communities were to emerge as beacons of resilience and resourcefulness. Over the years in which Leicester had been steadily earning its reputation as a testbed for multiculturalism, it had accumulated what might have come to be described as 'spiritual capital'. Now was the time to deploy this intangible but fruitful resource for the benefit not only of the communities themselves, but also of the city at large.

Leicester City Council, Leicestershire County Council and Rutland County Council formed a joint Faiths Engagement Group; I was one of a handful of officers from the three local authorities charged with running it. Colleagues from Public Health, the police and other agencies met regularly online with influential members of the local faith and cultural communities, staying abreast of the changing situation, sharing relevant data, information and statistics, obtaining an overall view of community needs, as well as surveying what they had to offer. The Faiths Engagement Group focused on practical matters related to life – and death – among local communities. As conditions changed, a team of city council officers visited places of worship to ensure compliance with government guidance as they started to reopen. As a member of that team, I saw at close quarters the rapacious impact of Covid-19 on the finances, premises, resources and morale of our communities. I was also involved in devising solutions to their difficulties, as well as ways of maximizing their assets to aid recovery. Places of worship became focal points for collection, consolidation and dispersal of food, clothing and medicines; arranged call rotas and doorstep visits to isolated and vulnerable people in their neighbourhoods; supported Mutual Aid Groups and other local efforts of good will. Colleagues who had previously been dismissive of the role of the faith communities in public life revised their opinion when they saw the positive impact they were able to make.

Leicester's agonizingly slow emergence from extended lockdown presented a fluid situation that required all involved to be light on their feet. I was but one of a sizeable team drawn from a range of public bodies involved in these efforts. I engaged with the faith and cultural communities here as fully as I could, while also bearing in mind the need to remain detached. There would have been no merit whatsoever in pushing my faith community or identity to the fore, or claiming undeserved credit for what was a widespread collective effort. Yet I am convinced that the involvement of even one Bahá'í definitely made a difference, not least through commitment to unity first and foremost – in this context entailing the harmony of religions and the necessity of an equitable approach to their communities and congregations.

In doing my best to do the right thing by everyone involved, I looked to the model of 'Abdu'l-Bahá (1844–1921) as 'the embodiment of every Bahá'í ideal, the incarnation of every Bahá'í ideal, the incarnation of every Bahá'í virtue [...] the Mainspring of the oneness of Humanity' (Shoghi Effendi, 1991, 134). Whenever my services were required, I asked myself – as all Bahá'ís would – 'What would 'Abdu'l-Bahá do?'

In the privacy of my chamber

According to 'Abdu'l-Bahá, 'There are no solitaries and no hermits among the Bahá'ís' ('Abdu'l-Bahá, 1982: 93). Lockdown made us feel like solitaries and hermits though, to varying degrees. Bahá'ís are no strangers to certain kinds of isolation. We are few in number and thinly spread, so it is not unusual for someone to be the only Bahá'í in their household, their place of work or study, even their city, town or village. One Bahá'í living somewhere without benefit of a local Bahá'í community is recognized as an 'isolated believer'. Lockdown forced on us a more extreme version of something with which Bahá'ís were already familiar. It also linked directly into the long-form narrative of the Bahá'í Faith, part of the shared *mythos* that binds members of our community together.

The three central figures of the Bahá'í Faith were subject to lengthy periods of incarceration, from house arrest to more formal imprisonment. 'Abdu'l-Bahá wrote of his father, Bahá'u'lláh, that 'He spent twenty-five long years in confinement and was insulted and tormented' ('Abdu'l-Bahá, 2021, 12.3). 'His one and only purpose in accepting such trials and tribulations for His blessed Self was to instruct the lovers in the ways of love and teach the longing souls the art of servitude' ('Abdu'l-Bahá 2021, 12.3, 30.3). Towards the end of his life, Bahá'u'lláh was visited by the English orientalist Edward Granville Browne, to whom he said, 'Thou hast come to see a prisoner and an exile' (Bahá'u'lláh, quoted in Esslemont, 1987, 39). The image of prison and prisoners applies not just to the history of our faith; it extends to understanding our place in the world. In *The Hidden Words*, Bahá'u'lláh advises, 'Free thyself from the fetters of this world, and loose thy soul from the prison of self' (Bahá'u'lláh, 2002, Part II. – From the Persian, 40). During collective lockdown and individual isolation, Bahá'ís were able to find comfort and inspiration in how the Báb, Bahá'u'lláh and 'Abdu'l-Bahá bore, endured and overcame their own periods of captivity, and how such a blunt instrument was unable to dim their light or silence their voices.

Being instructed to stay at home, even isolation, would not necessarily impact greatly on the spiritual practice of the individual Bahá'í. Bahá'u'lláh set the tone for our devotional life: 'Whoso reciteth, in the privacy of his chamber, the verses revealed by God, the scattering angels of the Almighty shall scatter abroad the fragrance of the words uttered by his mouth, and shall cause the heart of every righteous man to throb' (Bahá'u'lláh, 1991, iv). In terms of daily practice, every adult Bahá'í is expected to choose one of three different Obligatory Prayers revealed by Bahá'u'lláh; to read some portion of the Bahá'í writings morning and evening; and to recite the 'Greatest Name' (i.e. *Alláh'u'Abhá* – 'God Is the Most Glorious') ninety-five times once a day. There is a nineteen-day-long period of fasting in the month of March, when adult Bahá'ís in good health abstain from eating and drinking between sunrise and sunset (occurring once during lockdown). This is also framed as a personal responsibility, in which the individual is accountable only to God.

Bahá'ís have considerable agency and autonomy in how we express our faith in our lives, within certain clearly defined and widely understood guard rails:

> The Bahá'í teachings emphasize that each person is in charge of his or her own spiritual development. While institutions exist to guide and release energies, and Bahá'í community life is to be characterized by an atmosphere of cordial consultation and encouragement, the responsibility for spiritual growth ultimately rests with each individual. Indeed, there is no clergy in the Bahá'í Faith; the Bahá'í community can neither be described in terms of a pastor and congregation, nor as that of a body of believers led by learned individuals endowed with authority to interpret scriptures.
>
> (Bahá'í World Centre 2022)

This does not give us leeway to pick and choose from a menu of beliefs, principles and practices as we please. Such a blending of individual freedom with personal responsibility acknowledges a level of spiritual maturity and lends itself to a variety of settings, including the restrictions and opportunities arising from the pandemic.

The Bahá'í writings are central to spiritual development, both individual and collective. Bahá'u'lláh instructs us to 'Immerse yourselves in the ocean of My words, that ye may unravel its secrets, and discover all the pearls of wisdom that lie hid in its depths' (Bahá'u'lláh, 1992, 182). In lockdown, Bahá'í communities and institutions took advantage of widespread digital access and the prevalence of social media, tailoring presentations of the Bahá'í writings (as well as the principles and teachings that arise from them) to the needs of the hour across a range of platforms. Examples which I found personally beneficial include 'Elevate' (a curated anthology of accessible and thought-provoking quotations and talking points from Bahá'í and other sources to help raise the tone of discussion, reflection and action); 'Meaningful Conversations' (in which local Bahá'í communities hosted round-table discussions based on Bahá'í texts of relevance to the moment) and 'Studio Sessions' (video recordings of musical performances of extracts from the Bahá'í writings). These (and others) proved so popular and successful that they are enjoying life beyond lockdown.

Of course, Bahá'ís have collective gatherings for worship among other purposes. Foremost among these is the 19-Day Feast, held on the first day of each Bahá'í month. The Feast, as well as the nine Holy Days observed annually, were held online from the start of lockdown till well past its lifting. This had benefits as well as drawbacks. My work for the past fifteen years had often kept me busy in the evening and at weekends. Freed from such responsibilities, I took part in more Bahá'í community meetings during lockdown than I had in ages. I also participated in conferences, courses and webinars hosted by a variety of agencies, bodies and institutions that helped make lockdown a time of learning and growth for me.

Moving beyond Covid-19

The Bahá'í teachings say that difficulties, trials and suffering are unavoidable. From a spiritual perspective, they are drivers of individual and collective change, growth and progress – but only if they are recognized as such and the opportunities they offer are taken in that spirit. 'When all humanity is in the throes of dire suffering, the Bahá'ís should not hope to remain unaffected. [...] Such world crisis is necessary to awaken us to the importance of our duty and the carrying on of our task. Suffering will increase our energy in setting before humanity the road to salvation, it will move us from our repose' (Shoghi Effendi, 1931). In the face of suffering on the scale of the pandemic, Bahá'ís are more likely to ask what insights can be gained, what lessons can we learn about living together better. Rather than wonder, 'What kind of God would let this happen?', we are more likely to wonder what kind of people we are that, in possession of a super-abundance of advice, direction and guidance, we lurch from one crisis to the next, testing our institutions and relationships, with ever more damaging repercussions for those least able to bear the strain. Dipping into Bahá'u'lláh's *Hidden Words* once again, he says there, 'My calamity is my providence, outwardly it is fire and vengeance, but inwardly it is light and mercy' (Bahá'u'lláh, 2002, Part I. – From the Arabic, 51). At the very least, the pandemic prompted us to look in the mirror, to interrogate the motives for our actions, to consider our responsibilities to each other – to imagine other ways of being human. But to what extent will that stick, as the immediate dangers of Covid-19 recede from the headlines? 'No one is safe till everyone is safe' made for a great soundbite; is that all it will turn out to be?

As cautious as I might feel about speaking for my fellow Bahá'ís, I am confident in saying that we are not interested in returning to normal. 'Normal' included an awful lot of things that led to the pandemic in the first place and aggravated its effects. And whatever the 'new normal' is supposed to be, it looks a lot like the old normal, only more so. Bahá'ís were committed to big changes in the world before Covid-19. The pandemic has turned a spotlight on many topics where Bahá'ís have long been vocal and active: economic justice; equality of women and men; global governance; harmony of science and religion; unfettered investigation of truth; the value of work performed in the spirit of service; and elimination of prejudice. These are at the foundation of contemporary public discourse. Bahá'ís are under no illusion about the difficulties of the task ahead, but we are eager to engage in open and honest conversations, leading to positive action and genuine transformation. The pandemic is far from over – for the increasing numbers living with Long Covid, for those countries, nations, states where vaccines are in short supply, for those wary of the emergence of a new variant. If we really do want to make positive change that will ameliorate the continuing impact of Covid-19 and prepare us for whatever challenges come next, we commend to all well-wishers of humanity Bahá'u'lláh's pertinent instruction: 'Let your vision be world-embracing, rather than confined to your own self' (Bahá'u'lláh, 2005, 43.5).

References

'Abdu'l-Bahá. (1982). '*Abdu'l-Bahá in London*. London: Bahá'í Publishing Trust.

'Abdu'l-Bahá. (2021). *Light of the World: Selected Tablets of 'Abdu'l-Bahá*, trans. Shoghi Effendi et al. Haifa: Bahá'í World Centre.

Bahá'í World Centre. 'What Bahá'ís Do: Walking a Spiritual Path'. on The Bahá'í Faith: The Official Website of the Worldwide Bahá'í community. Accessible online at URL: https://www.bahai.org/action/response-call-bahaullah/walking-spiritual-path.

Bahá'u'lláh et al. (1991). *Bahá'í Prayers: A Selection of Prayers Revealed by Bahá'u'lláh, the Báb, and 'Abdu'l-Bahá*, trans. Shoghi Effendi et al. Wilmette: Bahá'í Publishing Trust.

Bahá'u'lláh. (1992). *The Kitáb-i-Aqdas: The Most Holy Book*, trans. Shoghi Effendi et al. Haifa: Bahá'í World Centre.

Bahá'u'lláh. (2002). *The Hidden Words*, trans. Shoghi Effendi with the assistance of some English friends. Wilmette, IL: Bahá'í Publishing.

Bahá'u'lláh. (2005). *Gleanings from the Writings of Bahá'u'lláh*, trans. Shoghi
    Effendi. Wilmette, IL: Bahá'í Publishing.
Esslemont, J. E. (1987). *Bahá'u'lláh and the New Era*, 5th rev. ed. (Wilmette:
    Bahá'í Publishing Trust.
Shoghi Effendi. From a letter written on behalf of Shoghi Effendi to an individual
    believer in reply to a letter dated 14 October 1931: *Bahá'í News*, January
    1932, 1.
Shoghi Effendi. (1991). *The World Order of Bahá'u'lláh: Selected Letters*.
    Wilmette, IL: Bahá'í Publishing Trust.

18

Jains and Covid-19

Vinod Kapashi

Introduction

Neil Armstrong, when he set foot on the moon, said, 'That's one small step for man, one giant leap for mankind.' Using these words in a different context, humankind has not seen any bigger or greater disaster in our recent past than the disaster caused by the Coronavirus. One small, invisible virus or one small mistake has resulted in one giant of a disaster throughout the world.

Over six hundred million people worldwide have had Covid-19 at the time of writing, and over 6.5 million people have died. However, these figures may be underestimates since some people did not notify the authorities or the doctors. In many cases, doctors certified that the death has occurred due to other underlying causes, and some governments may not have disclosed the true figure of deaths. Some photographs of burning funeral pyres in India were circulated worldwide by the media, alleging that that the government was hiding the true figures of the death toll. Whatever the true figures are, one thing is certain: Covid-19 has affected all of us on this globe, directly or indirectly.

Jains in the UK and in India

I am associated with many Jain organizations in the UK and know about one thousand Jain families. Each and every family is affected by Corona. Most of them have reported that a close relative, a friend or a friend of the friend had died due to Covid. Millions of people have suffered financial hardships due to lockdown imposed by the governments of many countries.

Jains are very much in the minority – there are only around 45,000 Jains in the UK, and six million worldwide – and some people even do not know that there is a religion called Jainism. We all have suffered greatly during the lockdown, which caused immense hardship for many families. Those who were earning wages by doing manual work and especially those who are daily wage earners suffered much hardship since they relied on day-to-day income for their basic needs and could not go out and work. They experienced a total loss of their earnings and found it very difficult to feed their families, and even found that there was no money for medicines or hospital treatment. In extreme cases, some had no money even for funerals. Most Western countries provided financial assistance to all those who were in dire needs. Many countries provided free medical help to those who were affected by the virus and were very ill.

In India, ordinary Jains suffered greatly due to Covid-19. Shops, schools, offices and factories were closed. There are no social security payments in India. Closure of shops meant total loss of income. Factories were closed too, and workers were made redundant or sacked. Workers on construction sites not only lost their jobs, but were left homeless. Jains, by and large, are business people or have positions with good salaries, affording a relatively comfortable lifestyle. However, those with large families suffered more heavily. No one has been able to combat these indirect effects of Covid-19: prices of essential commodities have increased greatly, and people are struggling to pay their bills. The war in Ukraine has added to worldwide inflation and hardship. All these effects are felt throughout the globe, irrespective of any distinction of race or religion.

A Jain view

So how have Jains viewed the situation and tried to cope with this calamity? Jainism, the ancient religion of India, has taught many principles to humankind. One very important principle mentioned by the Jain scriptures is 'reverence for all life'. When Jainism talks about 'life', it possesses the very first scripture to claim that there is life in the plants, in water, in air, on and below the earth and even in fire (Kapashi 1996). They feel pain when disturbed or hurt. The Jain monk Umaswatiji expresses his concern for looking after our environment in his book the *Tattvärtha Sutra*, in which he writes a famous aphorism *Parspropgraho Jeevana*, meaning that all life is interdependent (Doshi 2007: 89). We can only survive if we look after air, water, earth and other lives on this earth. We can only survive if we maintain a balance and harmony in nature. Many Jains – and also non-Jains – believe that natural disasters and diseases are the result of revenge by Mother Nature. It is the ruthless pursuit of industrial development; it is the greedy exploitations of resources; it is the manipulation of natural harmony; and it is the total disregard for animal sanctity that has caused the great imbalance. The clear result is global warming, droughts and the spread of viruses, which we all can see and feel. Some Jain monks have explained this in a different way: it is our karma. They have said that we have forgotten what was taught by Lord Mahavir, the twenty-fourth and last tirthankara of Jains. (A tirthankara is a teacher and saviour, one of whom appears in each successive aeon.) The Jain monks claim that we have committed misdeeds for which we are now being punished.

What Mahavir said was endorsed by Mahatma Gandhi: There is enough for everyone's need but there is not enough for everyone's greed. Even Jains have forgotten their important precept called *aparigraha* or non-possessiveness. We buy, we accumulate, and we increasingly discard material things. Continuous lockdown taught many Jains to stop going on a spending spree and to be satisfied with limited possessions. Whatever the cause of Covid-19, it has brought the highflying men and women down to earth and has shown them the real meaning of life and death. Jain religion has advised us to observe some very simple tenets, such as 'Do not acquire more than you really need and do not harm nature'. Jainism helps to live a balanced and healthy life. For good health, one should drink boiled water and avoid eating after sunset, look after other needy and sick people, wear a mouth-covering, keep social distance and not shake hands when greeting someone. The Jain scripture *Ogh Niryukti* provides guidelines about how to keep away from people who have contagious diseases and how to treat them (Deepratna 2009: 191). Readers may be familiar with Jain monks and nuns who wear face-coverings all the time. The Jain teachers advocated this hundreds of years ago, and it is practised widely. Ordinary people greet each other with Namaste or Jai Jinendra – respectful greetings which do not involve shaking hands. *Ogh Niryukti* also mentions washing hands and maintaining social distancing.

The effect of Covid on Jains

As soon as the lockdown was announced, places of worship were closed down, as well as community halls where regular lectures and cultural events were held. Closure of Jain temples meant that it became very difficult to carry on with essential religious rituals, as prescribed in the Jain texts. Priests and religious workers could not visit the temples to perform their routine tasks. This was considered unacceptable in many circles, but worshippers had no option, and almost every temple in the UK and in India saw a big decline in donations. Donation boxes in the temples were almost empty. Community halls, which were regularly hired out to members for their private gatherings, experienced big financial losses. I know two large Jain organizations in the UK who have built very large halls with ample parking facilities, and which lay empty for more than two years. One organization suffered heavy losses, but the other managed to convince the health authorities to open a vaccination centre in their premises.

Most Jain organizations in the UK started showing worship rituals on YouTube regularly. These became quite popular within few months, and for some it was even more convenient. The Mahavir Foundation (MF) is just one example in the UK which started showing daily *aarti* ritual on YouTube. MF has devised a scheme whereby whoever books the *aarti* has his or her name announced before the start of the ritual. MF started receiving a few names every day. Some even thought it was a better idea to see the *aarti* virtually rather than remain present at the temple premises. Birthdays and other events were celebrated with the names of the donors by booking an *aarti* ritual. MF has continued this practice even though there are no lockdown measures now because it was popular, and also brings revenue. As the community halls were all shut, religious discourses were also broadcast via Zoom and YouTube.

Compassion in Jainism

The concept of *Jeevdaya* in Jainism is important in this context. *Jeevdaya* is compassion towards all living beings. All Jain trusts and temples have *Jeevdaya* funds. Not only did they all have some money: some of the monks made special appeals to all Jains to donate generously and pay into Covid Relief funds. Millions of rupees were raised in India. One Jain trust run by a monk called Ratnasundarsuri has a large number of volunteers who have helped the poor by distributing food, clothing and cash. The revered monk Namramuni opened many religious shelters for the sick people. Food and medicines were given to all. Jains also run many animal sanctuaries called *panjarapoles*. Thousands of sick and aged animals are kept and looked after until they die. Jains donate millions of rupees every year to these *panjarapoles*. The animals' needs increased during the Covid period, but Jains managed to provide for all of them.

During the lockdown, I conducted a survey for an organization called Navjivan Vadil Kendra in the UK. This organization serves senior citizens of Harrow, Wembley, Barnet and Hillingdon areas. A number of questionnaires were sent to the members and one hundred (out of about 350) replies were received, mostly from the Jain families.

Seventy-three per cent of replies were from the people above seventy years. Forty per cent were doing walking exercises of about a kilometre every day, mostly indoors. However, what was interesting was that 95 per cent of participants were practising yoga and *pranayam* (breathing exercises), suggesting that people became slightly less reliant on doctors' prescriptive medicines. People were also asked about shopping problems. Eighty-four per cent said that their children or neighbours were shopping on their behalf, and the remaining 16 per cent did their own shopping locally. All of the respondents were in touch with relatives by phone or social media. An important question was about disappointment and depression during this difficult time. No one felt that they were depressed or were extremely unhappy, although 30 per cent said that they felt lonely, bored and somewhat disappointed because they were missing their usual outings and programmes. Seventy per cent said that they were not disappointed at all as they found things to do in the house like cleaning the house, learning how to cook new dishes, gardening, reading, watching television and of course attending meetings on Zoom. Most of these senior citizens now know how to use the internet for their contacts and hearing lectures and music.

What we have learned

The main change that has occurred is in people's attitudes and how they see life and death. We have realized that we are on this earth for a temporary spell only. Life is uncertain and death can strike at any time. Mahavir said to a disciple, 'A man's life does not last long and could end at any moment like a dew-drop sitting on the top of a blade of grass … which falls off in wind' (Kapashi 1996: 12). We have realized this during the pandemic.

We have learned quite a few things. We must donate our money and our time for good causes. We must help fellow human beings and we must understand other people's needs too. One thing has struck us all: we all are equal. There should not be any discrimination on the grounds of race, religion or gender. After all, the natural calamities do not make any such distinction!

References

Deepratna, M. S. (2009). *Ogh Niryukti*. (Gujarati version). Ahmedabad, India: Shrut Ratnakar.
Doshi, Manu (trans.) (2007). *Tattvärtha Sutra*. Ahmedabad, India: Shrut Ratnakar.

Kapashi, Vinod. (1996). *In Search of the Ultimate*. Ahmedabad, India: Mahavir
  Foundation.
World Health Organization. (2022). Coronavirus Disease (COVID-19) Pandemic.
  Accessible online at URL: https://www.who.int/emergencies/diseases/novel-
  coronavirus-2019.

19

Jain perceptions of the pandemic

Kumarpal Desai

Explanations

No event in human history has created so much havoc in so short a time than Covid-19 and its worldwide spread. The first case of Corona was reported on 17 November 2019 in Wuhan, China, and the virus spread to most countries and continents in less than fifty days. At that time, Jainism, known as a religion of non-violence, regarded the situation as a result of the killing of animals by human beings. In Jainism, non-violence is considered as the ultimate religious principle, and violence is considered the root of all evils and sorrows. The great Indian scholar Umaswati (first to fifth century CE – dates uncertain) taught that each life is based on the life of another, teaching us the most basic value of harmony with nature. Perhaps Covid-19 is the result of ignoring and blatantly violating this principle.

The principles of Jainism

In the past, animals and birds have been banished from their natural habitats and their natural life has been taken away. So the loss of their natural life has caused the spread of the virus by animals, such as mice, pigs and cows. The Jain religion consistently opposes the violent and cruel trading of wild animals, the mistreatment of animals on farms and transporting them for long distances. Jainism believes that the slaughter of any living being is equivalent to the slaughter of one's own soul. Jains believe that the virus was created due to animal slaughtering, thus changing the face of whole the world.

Covid-19 has compelled us to change our lifestyle and our daily religious practices. Jain organizations made extensive efforts to connect digitally with members of their community when collective, in-person celebrations and temple visits were either reduced in number, limited in capacity or cancelled because of the pandemic. While many passionately longed for their old practices, most Jains knew that they had no choice but to accept the findings of the scientists, and make changes in the interest of health and safety. Some seemingly unavoidable rituals had to be postponed. At first, people were not too concerned about the situation, but gradually they began to understand its seriousness. Some people who used to go to the temple every day to worship started using a sacred image in their house. Some temples offered small images to their worshippers so that they could worship at home, and those who wished to maintain their regular tradition of daily worship could continue their devotion.

Pandemics and other disasters are to be found in Jain scriptures, where invisible calamities like plague, influenza and famine have befallen human beings. Many Jain monks have faced such misfortunes. It is said that an epidemic had spread in the time of the learned monk Shri Bhadrabahu Swami (c. 433–c. 357 BCE?). At that time he composed the *Uvasaggaharan Stotra* – a prayer with poetic structure, which many people today recite – when they experience difficulties in life.

When the Spanish flu outbreak occurred in 1918, about eighteen million people died in India. This was the highest number of deaths in the world due to the negligence of the British government. Those who followed the Jain religion were therefore aware of such natural calamities, so instead of being terrified, they tried to comprehend it and reformed their religious activities accordingly.

Adaptations to rituals

Adaptations were made when the temples were closed, and religious ceremonies were suspended. However, in our religion, the soul, not the body, is glorified: here is much significance attached to self-knowledge and self-discovery. Since religion is focused on the soul, self-centred practices increased. At the same time, emphasis was given to contemplation. In addition, Jainism glorifies breathing meditation, and as Corona enters through the breath, so breathing exercises became more prevalent. Jain monks and nuns, who reside in their temples in separate apartments, could perform worship, and hence experienced no problems. Instead of monks and nuns going from house to house for their food during Covid-19, the Jain community made arrangements for their food. When temples were closed and hospitals were overcrowded, the temple arranged to provide free medicine made from herbs, and other natural treatments and homeopathic medicines. In addition, some Jain centres distributed food packages, and provided masks and ration kits.

Monks of two sects – Sthanakvasi and Terapanthi – and their sub-sects cover their mouths with a small cloth tied to the mouth. Other monks, on the other hand, keep a cloth called *muhpatti* in their hands discreetly during a conversation. The Jain monastic practice of keeping one's mouth covered helps to prevent the spread of bacteria and viruses, and hence mask-wearing did not present any problem. Additionally, there has been a rule of conduct for centuries about drinking boiled water, and a tradition of washing hands and feet entering someone's house. Monks and nuns observe fasting, and take a vow of eating two to four morsels less even if they are hungry, so there is control over one's diet. When they meet they join hands from a distance saying *Jai Jinendra*. The importance of all these religious matters was understood at the time of Covid-19.

Guidance from ancient scripture

Twenty-four hundred years ago there was an awareness of touch. The World Health Organization states that people infected with the virus should not be touched and that one should wear gloves if they need to be touched. Similar guidance is to be found in the scripture *Oghaniryukti*, written in the Middle Indo-Aryan Prakrit language: 'Whoever helps [the patient] to turn over, do not touch him directly, but only touch him after wrapping the cloth in his hand. It is also written that after turning the patient over, the hands must be washed with mud.' The text, which is written twenty-four hundred years ago, also mentions that the sick should be quarantined and kept in a separate house. If no separate room can be found in the house or if it is not possible to keep such distancing, a curtain should be hung in the house so that the victim may not come in contact with others, and transmission is lessened.

It is written in the same scripture, 'Do not touch the thing which is touched by the infected person and do not move from the door from which the sick person goes through it for his own actions.' Do not take food or water from the infected house, because it can increase the transmission. Never touch metal, as this can also increase the transmission. It was mentioned in the scripture years ago about isolation and social distance in dealing with an infected person. Thus, the rules and practices of the World Health Organization and other scientists for combating Covid-19 were anticipated by Jain monks, who came to know about viruses many years ago.

If we look at the adaptations that have taken place during the pandemic, they can be seen to maintain the original sentiments of the Jain religion. The popularity of online lectures instead of public lectures by monks has increased. Masks were distributed free of charge by the temples, while mass ceremonies, mass meals, horse-drawn carriages and ceremonies for breaking the fast were closed. For hundreds of years, the religion has celebrated its largest festival – Paryushan Parva. Even when India was governed by foreign rulers, and during the Mughal period, its observance did not stop. For the very first time the Corona virus caused the celebration to be stopped, and all accepted and complied. Pratikraman, a penitential ritual, usually involves lectures, city travel and a general spirit of devotion, but all these were banned, and remarkably no one insisted on celebrating. Pilgrimages to different sacred sites were forbidden, and Jains showed the ability and creativity to adjust to the situation.

Contemplation

Drastic changes were seen due to Covid-19. People began to think seriously about their own lives and started reflecting more about the importance of the soul. Due to the dreadful situation, compassion was aroused, and there was a desire to help other people more as people realized that their lives depended on others.

The pandemic changed the face of the world and made a tremendous revolution in human lifestyle, causing people to experience a state of isolation and loneliness. Leaders of the Jain Community had set up Mahajan – an organization dedicated to promoting education, offering medical aid and assistance for people's livelihood. This has enabled the rich to help people in times of disasters created by human beings or natural disasters. During the pandemic, no distinction of caste, creed, community or religion was observed in providing such assistance. In times of peace, the Mahajan used to dig step wells, wells and lakes. They established almonry and charity homes. Their philanthropic work was not exclusively done by Jains but involved other religions. More than 35,000 volunteers from the Jain Alert Group of India helped enormously during the pandemic time. They provided food, medicines and money to the needy. Free food packets were delivered far and wide, as well as grain and Indian traditional Ayurvedic herbs.

Three waves of Covid-19 have now ended, but Covid-19 has not been eradicated. At present when cases are on the rise in India, the pre-Covid world of religion has now changed completely. Self-satisfaction has given way to the courage to live in the midst of adversity. Although mobile phones could not previously be utilized, due to the lack of electricity in some places, the use of mass media has now become commonplace. However, restraint in the use of social media is advisable.

Public healthcare providers and health workers, who are in direct contact with Covid-19 patients, have increased their prestige everywhere. There is a growing sense of respect for doctors, nurses and other hospital staff who risk their lives to save others. However, the Jain religion continues to glorify spirituality, yoga and music in solitude, and to spread the religious feeling of living in peace with other living beings. The reliance on science during the pandemic has prompted human beings who were previously were superstitious to avoid prevalent superstitious practices and understand the disease from a scientific perspective. Stress and grief are recognized as anxiety disorders – Covid-19 syndrome and clinical depression. Nonetheless, religion plays a role in overcoming such conditions, and psychiatrists, together with writers and journalists have shown how religious teachings can be used to overcome such problems. The human mind tries to cultivate fearlessness by facing terror through religion.

Towards global unity

One of the key concepts of Jainism is global unity, regarding the entire human race as one. The Coronavirus has united humankind, and we have learned a lot from this pandemic. Human beings have emerged as the dominant species, but at the same time everyone has seen how a small virus can cause so much human misery, with the possible threat of other such viruses looming over humanity. All our advances in technology must now for the welfare of this earth and all need to think collectively. Let us make this earth a friendly abode with Jainism's key principles, which are non-violence, truth, non-possession and non-absolutism.

References

Bhadrabahu Swami. (2011). *Uvasaggaharan Stotra*. Mumbai: Parasdham.
Maes, Claire. (2022). 'Framing the Pandemic: An Examination of How WHO Guidelines Turned into Jain Religious Practices'. *Religions* 13: 377. https://doi.org/10.3390/ rel13050377. Accessible online at URL: https://www.mdpi.com/2077-1444/13/5/377/htm.

Oghaniryukti (ओघनिर्युक्ती) is a Jain text attributed to Bhadrabāhu.

Tattvārtha Sūtra. (ed. Vinod Kapashi, 1995). Accessible online at URL: https://www.jainfoundation.in/JAINLIBRARY/books/tattvartha_sutra_that_which_is_007758_std.pdf.

Wiley, Kristi L. (2004). *Historical Dictionary of Jainism.* Lanham, Toronto and Oxford: Scarecrow Press.

20

African religion: Vibrant amid Covid-19 in Eswatini

Hebron L. Ndlovu

The people of the Kingdom of Eswatini (formally Swaziland) are deeply religious. They are ruled by a sacred monarchy that is firmly attached to Swazi Religion while simultaneously openly embracing and commending the Christian faith. It is estimated that around two thirds of the Swazi are affiliated to various Christian churches while 33 per cent are committed adherents to Swazi Religion. There is also a small number of Swazi who affiliated to Islam and the Bahá'í Faith (Ndlovu 2014a).

I am a bona fide Swazi national and a Christian. I subscribe to the view that indigenous African Religion is a lived religion that co-exists with Christianity, Islam and other religions in sub-Saharan Africa (Olupona 2014). In the Kingdom of Eswatini, Swazi Religion (the indigenous African Religion of Eswatini) is very much alive and vibrant; and its key doctrines are preserved and communicated through annual rituals such as Incwala ritual of kingship (Ndlovu 2011).

Annual Christian ceremonies in Eswatini in the pre-Covid-19 era

Christian churches, as I observed elsewhere (Ndlovu 2014b: 274), enjoy special privileges vis-à-vis other faith communities in the country. They are permitted, for example, to proselytize over national radio and television stations, and Christian prayers are said in public schools and offices and at national ceremonies. The dominance of the Christian religion in Swazi society is most noticeable during annual national festivals and ceremonies such as Good Friday, Somhlolo Festival of Praise and Beginning of Year/End of Year Royal Christian Services. At these ceremonies, the Swazi monarchy implores the nation to embrace the Christian faith despite the fact the sacred monarchy itself is not formally attached to any Christian church (Ndlovu 2014b; Ndlovu 2019).

Coordinated by African Initiated Churches, the Good Friday ceremony is one of the main national ceremonies in the kingdom in which Swazi Christians celebrate Easter with the Ngwenyama, Indlovukazi and the nation. The services take place at the Ndlovukazi's residence at Ludzidzini, the National Church at Lobamba, the Ngwenyama's residence called Ngabezweni and the Somhlolo National Stadium. The Somhlolo Festival of Praise is coordinated by the evangelical churches but hosted by the Ndlovukazi. At this function King Somhlolo (who ruled over Eswatini from 1818 to 1836) is celebrated for inviting Christian missionaries to the Kingdom (Ndlovu 2014b).

The Beginning of Year and End of Year services, hosted by the Ngwenyama, are relatively new annual Christian Services that are held in January/February and November/December at Lozitha Palace to pray for the sacred monarchy and invoke God's guidance and blessing as the year begins and ends, respectively. The climax of both ceremonies involves sermons given by the Ndlovukazi and the Ngwenyama (Ndlovu 2019).

Annual ceremonies of Swazi religion

The depiction of the numerical dominance of the Christian religion should not mislead the reader into thinking that African Religion is less significant compared to Christianity. Most Africans in sub-Saharan Africa identify themselves as Christian while they simultaneously uphold the main doctrines and practices of African Religion (Maluleke 2010; Olupona 2014; Ndlovu 2014b). Likewise, the indigenous annual ceremonies carry equal, if not more, weight than the annual Christian ceremonies described above. Three annual indigenous ceremonies are particularly noteworthy: Umhlanga (the Reed Dance), Buganu (the Marula wine festival) and Incwala (the sacred Kingship ceremony). All three national functions revolve around the sacred dual monarchy of the Kingdom of Eswatini, namely Ingwenyama (the Lion King) and Indlovukazi (the She Elephant or the Queen Mother).

The Umhlanga (Reed Dance) is a colourful four-day ceremony held in August or September to honour and pay tribute to the Ndlovukazi as a sacred monarch. At this function multitudes (in 2015 about 100,000) of young, unmarried women from all regions walk long distances to collect fresh reeds, carry the heavy bundles to the Ndlovukazi's residence at Ludzidzini. The maidens deliver the reed to the queen mother to use as a windbreak, and sing and dance before her, the king and more than 20,000 spectators (Ndlovu 2014b). The climax of ceremony is the last day (which effectively becomes a public holiday) in which the maidens normally dance topless before the king and the queen mother; and they wear colourful traditional mini-skirts. On behalf of the nation, the Ngwenyama demonstrates his appreciation by performing a giya dance and placing his cow shield before each regimental group. The festival promotes such dominant cultural values as virginity, resourcefulness, social responsibility and loyalty to the monarchy (Ndlovu 2014b).

Buganu ceremony is a national marula-wine festival that is held in February/March in honour of the Ndlovukazi at her rural residences situated at Buhleni and Hlane northeast of Swaziland. The ceremony celebrates motherhood and the gift of life through the marula-fruit harvest; and it is characterized by feasting, song, dance and fellowship. At this ceremony the Lutsango (a group of all adult Swazi mothers) bring along large quantities (at least twenty litres each) of fresh wine made from wild marula fruit. Thousands of mothers from the four regions of the country bring their traditional brew. Three main standardized activities characterize the Buganu festival: feasting and drinking; song and dance and brief speeches by the Ndlovukazi and the Ngwenyama.

The Incwala ceremony is the most sacred annual ceremony of Swazi Religion. It is both a celebration of the first fruits of summer harvest and sacred kingship. Hosted by the Indlovukazi at her residence at Ludzidzini, the Ncwala affords the Ngwenyama the privilege to present the nation's prayers to God through the national ancestors (Ndlovu 2011). All Swazi are expected to participate in the ceremony, wearing their indigenous Incwala attire. Christians also participate in the ceremony. Some leaders of the African indigenous churches prefer to represent their churches formally at the Incwala, wearing their clerical robes. Over the years, the leaders of the indigenous churches have not only been dancing the Incwala, but they have been praying for the success of the Incwala every year (Ndlovu 2019).

The impact of Covid on annual ceremonies

Beginning in March 2020, Covid-19 dealt a heavy blow on all the known Swazi national religious ceremonies since all gatherings of more than twenty people were prohibited. This followed a Declaration of National Emergency which was accompanied by numerous Coronavirus regulations that were enforced by, among others, security forces, police, chiefs, community police and personnel engaged by the government Department of Health. The core message encapsulated by the regulations was that people had to limit their movement, stay at home and leave home only when it was absolutely necessary. Major national ceremonies were either cancelled altogether or severely downscaled in terms of number of participants.

National Christian ceremonies

In 2020 and 2021, the Good Friday ceremony, in which normally the king and queen mother hosted thousands of Christians at different venues, could only have at least twenty persons converging in one single venue at the National Church. Even then, the duration of every public religious ceremony could not exceed two hours. In 2020 the late prime minister (Mr Mandvulo Dlamini who succumbed to Covid-19 complications in November 2020) urged every Christian to stay at home and assured the nation at 'Our National Good Friday and Easter Services will be broadcast live on television and radio with a link on Government social media platforms to allow all EmaSwati, in and out of the country, to access them' (Government of the Kingdom of Swatini [2020]).

Indeed, during the Good Friday of 2020, the Ngwenyama and the Ndlovukazi were not present, but were represented by the Royal Governor, the prime minister, senior princess and princesses, selected cabinet ministers and members of parliament. Christians were represented by the leaders of the country's three main church organizations: Eswatini Conference of Churches, Council of Churches in Swaziland and the League of African Churches in Africa. Prominent church leaders who participated at the historic Good Friday of 2020 included the late Bishop Stephen Masilela (president of the Eswatini Conferences of Churches who succumbed to a Covid-19-related illness later in 2020), the late Bishop Elizabeth Wamukowa (Bishop of the Anglican Church who also died from a Covid-related sickness), Bishop Jose Luis Gerrado Ponce de Leon of the Catholic Church of Eswatini and Bishop Samson Hlatshwako, president of the League of African Churches in Africa. All participants had to wear face masks even when preaching and singing.

Another national Christian ceremony that was held during the Covid era was Somhlolo Festival of Praise. As with the Good Friday Ceremony, the Covid regulations were upheld tenaciously. The Ngwenyama, royalty, government and churches were duly represented. The ceremony was broadcast live on national television and radio. However, the Beginning of Year and End of Year Celebrations which were normally held at Lozitha Palace were never held during the Covid-19 period.

National indigenous ceremonies

Although the three indigenous national ceremonies described previously (Umhlanga, Buganu and Incwala) are significant, in 2020 and 2021 Buganu ceremony was cancelled completely. It was only Umhlanga and Incwala that were moderately performed, and in different ways.

The Umhlanga ceremonies of 2020 and 2021 were miniature functions in the true sense of the word. A smaller group of maidens not exceeding 200, and representing different regions in the kingdom converged at Ludzidzini royal residence to cut the reed and present it to the queen mother. There were fewer than one hundred spectators. All the maidens and observers had to wear face masks, and everyone had to be screened for Covid prior to joining the ceremony. The ceremony was broadcast live on national television and radio for the benefit of multitudes of Swazi men and women who could not attend the function because of Covid restrictions. Nonetheless, the number of participants at the Umhlanga exceeded the stipulated minimum number of twenty by far.

When it came to Incwala ceremonies, the known Covid restrictions pertaining to number of participants were further suspended. In 2020 when the nation was invited through national television and radio to participate in the ceremony, no restriction on numbers was made except that participants had to be representative of different regions of the country, and that every participant had to pass the Covid test, wear a mask and sanitize before they could take part. In his own words, the Governor of Ludzidzini royal residence where the main performances of Incwala take place urged the nation as follows:

> People cannot be stopped from participating in cultural events, The ceremony goes on and all people are expected to attend in numbers. I hope things will go back to normal after the pandemic … Warriors will be expected to follow instructions from the Ministry of Health, No one is expected to go against the instructions.
>
> (Shange 2020)

Indeed, thanks to the Ministry of Health that regulated the flow of people into the Sibaya (the Cattle Byre in which Incwala is performed), the Incwala of 2020 was hailed by Sibusiso Shange of the *Times of Swaziland* as a success: 'EmaSwati yesterday successfully celebrated the annual Incwala Ceremony despite the striking Covid-19 pandemic' (Shange 2021). However, the Incwala of 2020 did not conclude in the normal way. Ordinarily the formal end of Incwala happens after the formal dismissal of the regiment by the king following the mandatory Imfabantfu or the Weeding of Royal Fields (Ndlovu 2011).

Conclusion

Although Covid-19 impacted negatively on normal operations of the Christian faith and African Religion, the latter faith tradition was less affected. What we observe about the apparent primacy of African Religion in the actual lives of the Swazi – who collectively define themselves as a Christian nation – cannot be seen as entirely unique in the Kingdom of Eswatini. Rather, it appears to be a pointer to the fact that for many (if not most) Africans, the indigenous worldviews, beliefs and values reign supreme in the hearts and minds of the people amid Covid; and despite the thin veil of modernity sweeping across sub-Saharan Africa.

References

Government of the Kingdom of Swatini. (2020). *Press Statement, Office of the Prime Minister*. 20 March. Mbabane: Eswatini.

Maluleke, T. (2010). 'Of Africanised Bees and Africanised Churches: Ten Theses on African Christianity'. *Missionalia* 38 (3): 369–80.

Ndlovu, H. L. (2002). 'Positive Images of Women in Swazi Traditional Religion'. *UNESWA Research Journal* 16 (December), 19–25.

Ndlovu, H. L. (2011). 'Swazi Religion and the Environment: The Case of the Ncwala Ritual'. *BOLESWA Journal of Theology, Religion and Philosophy* 1 (3): 116–34.

Ndlovu, H. L. (2014a). 'Christian Identity amid African Religion: *Buganu* Ceremony and the Construction of Multiple Religious Identities in Swaziland' in *Christian Identity and Justice in a Globalized World from a Southern African Perspective*. H. Kroesbergen ed., Wellington, South Africa: Christian Literature Fund (CLF).

Ndlovu, H. L. (2014b). 'Swaziland'. In. T. Riggs, ed., *Worldmark Encyclopedia of Religious Practices* Vol. 4, 2nd edn, Farmington, MI: Gale: 273–85.

Ndlovu, H. L. (2019). 'Joint Worship Ceremonies of Africanists and Christians in the Kingdom of Swaziland'. In Cohn-Sherbok, Dan and Lewis, Christopher eds., *Interfaith Worship and Prayer: We Must Pray Together*. London: Jessica Kingsley Publishers.

Olupona, J. K. (2014). 'African Traditional Religion', In Riggs, T., ed., *Worldmark Encyclopedia of Religious Practices,* vol. 1, 2nd edn, Farmington, MI: Gale: 1–23.

Shange, Sibusiso. (2020). 'Everyone Is Invited to Incwala-King'. *Times of Swaziland*. 14 December 2020. Accessible online at URL: http://www.times. co.sz/news/131150-everyone-is-invited-to-incwala-king-html.

Shange, Sibusiso. (2021). 'Incwala Ceremony a Success Despite Covid-19 Era'. *Times of Swaziland*. 3 January 2021. Accessible online at URL: http://www. times.co.sz/news/131312-incwala-ceremony-a-success-despite-covid-19-era-html.

Swaziland Government. (2005). *The Constitution of the Kingdom of Swaziland*. Swaziland, Mbabane.

21

Opening our eyes: Covid-19 and indigenous funeral processes in African Traditional Religion

Nokuzola Mndende

Introduction

The arrival of the Coronavirus in the country, like all other pandemics, was interpreted in many ways, either caused by natural phenomena or chemical warfare or wrath of the ancestors for the people's misdeeds. From an African Traditional Religion (ATR) perspective, funerals had been the most affected due to government regulations. Due to the nature of the religion and the effects of the pandemic, it will be important to first give a brief introduction about the faith and a specific area mostly affected.

The effects of Covid-19 have changed the practice of ATR in South Africa in both the negative and positive ways. Since the practice of African culture and spirituality that we have today has been affected by colonialism and the introduction of Christianity most Blacks became nominal Christians which means that they did not abandon their culture and indigenous spirituality but also professed Christianity. This affected the way they conducted their rituals which became a mixture of ATR and Christianity. This is important to mention in this chapter because in most funerals Black Christians include some new practices like night vigils and an almost-whole-day service which cause some grey areas in the religious practices.

In discussing this topic it will also be useful to first briefly unpack· the understanding of death within the indigenous African community in context. To avoid generalization, I will focus on the effects of the pandemic amongst the Xhosa communities who are residing in both rural and urban areas.

In an African context the concept of a nuclear family in isolation from the extended family does not exist. Each individual is defined by the genealogy he or she comes from, and this includes the living and the departed, the ancestors. It is believed that these departed members of the family are also intermediaries between the Creator and the living. As a result of this aspect amongst the basic beliefs in ATR, the living always keep this unwavering relationship intact. In all the rituals performed, ancestors play a crucial role for the success of each ritual.

Due to migrant labour and urbanization, many families have partially moved from rural areas to the cities. Many of these families have two residents, one in rural areas and one in the cities, but the one in the rural areas is regarded as *ikhaya* ('home') where rituals are performed and where one is expected to be buried. Because of this problem of living in two worlds, that is, the city and the rural, when one passes on in the city, there are some additional ritual performances that are done by members of the family before taking the body home to the rural areas. It is important to mention these as they had been seriously affected by the impact of Covid-19. These are summarized as follows.

Stage 1: Dying far from home

When a person dies outside home, whether in hospital or by accident somewhere out of home, before the body is taken home, he or she must be taken to the place where the soul left the body. A member of the family must 'inform' the deceased and tell him or her that this is the place where his or her spirit left the body and they have now come to take spirit home. The belief is that after the accident the spirit will be still hovering around the place of the accident and it needs to be 'taken' home. If not done it is believed that it will remain there and that could cause problems to his or her offspring. Non-performance of this act will definitely lead to another ritual to be performed later to take him or her home spiritually, *ukumlanda ngokomoya*. To avoid all this, the body is taken, as said earlier, to the point where death occurred, then to the residence where he or she was living. Again, in this place where he or she was residing, he or she will be told that this is his or her home where he or she stayed in the area, and now is being taken home to join his or her ancestors.

Stage 2: *Viewing the body*

Because these days people die away from home, or even if they die at home, the bodies do go to mortuaries and mix with other bodies, it is therefore compulsory that families make sure that they bury the right person. When a mortuary brings the body home the driver is always compelled to open the coffin so that the elderly members of the family could come and identify the body and be satisfied that they are burying the correct body.

Stage 3: *Number of attendees in a funeral*

Number of attendees in the funeral is not restricted. An understanding of family in Africa is different from the West. *Ikhaya* (home – consisting of family members) is the basic unit that constitutes the family. Mbiti (1969:104) refers to this structure as one which he calls 'kinship', and he regards it as an existing basic unit through blood and betrothal (marriage). In African tradition marriage is a union between two families and not between two people. These two families become one and they share joys and sorrows. If there is death, they come to share the sorrows and mourn together. Besides these family members mentioned above, one must not forget that each individual is living within a traditional community. All these make the numbers of people attending the funeral to increase, something which became problematic when Covid-19 regulations were imposed by the government.

Stage 4: *Putting a stone* (ukubeka ilitye)

In all funerals, family members are supposed to 'put a stone' on top of the grave which symbolizes that a person has now reached closure that a relative has passed on and it is where he or she is 'lying'. This is very necessary to the extent that even those who did not attend the funeral would come at a later stage to 'put the stone'.

Stage 5: Ukuseza/ukuphuza amanzi *(literally, 'drinking still water')*

Ukuseza/ukuphuza amanzi is a small ceremony normally performed a day after the funeral as a cleansing ceremony for those members of the family who will be departing to their respective homes. Few members of the community attend to admonish the mourners on how to behave after the loss of their member.

Stage 6: Ukuhlamba Iipeki *(cleansing of the utensils used in digging the grave)*

As in the rural areas, it is the young men who dig the grave using their picks and spades, which they normally leave at the homestead after digging, because they are regarded as unclean. A week after the funeral in some communities, a ritual of *Ukuhlamba iipeki* (cleansing of picks) is performed and they are then returned to their respective owners. Though this is not a big ceremony, but the male members of the community would come to the family and there is no restricted number of attendees because there is also African beer prepared, so there will be young and old males.

Meaning of death

From an African perspective, death does not mean the destruction of life; it is a transition stage before an individual can enter the world of ancestors. It marks the physical separation of the individual from this physical life and the joining of his or her soul with the spiritual world. Death does not only mark the transition to the spiritual world, but it also carries with it the obligation to look after the welfare of the living. It is an opening into another life – a continuation of the present one, so this communication continues.

As death is described as a transition stage en route to the world of the ancestors, the deceased person is mostly referred to metaphorically in some specific ways like 'he or she has gone, has disappeared, is no longer with us, is absent, or is somewhere'. Such references indicate that though an individual has left this world, he or she will keep on communicating with his or her people and will now be in a powerful position. Although the soul has departed from the flesh, his or her spiritual body is believed to still be composed of 'sensory' organs, hence a belief that the deceased can 'hear, see, touch, feel and occupy space'. This makes it clear that the last methods of putting the body of the deceased into the grave should be treated in a respectful manner. The bones of the deceased are also treated with great respect and are believed to have the ability to speak (*ayathetha*), to hear (*ayeva*) when someone is talking to them. This importance of 'bones' is a strong indication that in ATR cremation is tabooed.

Another important metaphor used in reference to human bones is *ayashukuma*, meaning that they can 'shake or move'. This 'vibration' of *amathambo* (of bones) means that they are believed to be responding to whatever situation that needs their intervention or response. When ancestors are angry, their wrath is associated with *ukushukuma kwamathambo* (shaking/vibration of the bones). Ignoring the consistent messages from the ancestors is believed to be one of the causes of some present catastrophes in the world, something that needs some form of correcting measures or appeasement. When a catastrophe attacks the community, there are several rules and regulations to appease and to mourn depending on the nature of the catastrophe. If all the above processes are not done, it is generally believed that the deceased may continue to punish those still living, especially relatives of the deceased person who ought to give the deceased a respectful funeral process and burial.

Looking at the above beliefs and practices, it will be important when dealing with the effects of Covid-19 that the focus should be on the affected beliefs and practices like banning of the viewing the body by family members, restricted number of attendees in funerals and banning of crucial rituals.

Covid-19 regulations

Government regulations involved some serious restrictions on the funeral processes and there were many conflicting impositions. As a result of these restrictions, the government was accused of being against African culture and spirituality, and anti-poor. Because the disease was regarded as highly contagious, family members were not allowed to view the body. As a result of this problem, it had been in the media (print and electronic) that many families buried wrong bodies, some learnt later that they had to exhume the graves because they had buried wrong bodies. Different stories from different families were very common during this era. One grieving woman, for example, said, 'They refused to allow me to view my husband's body at the hospital mortuary due to Covid-19 regulations. Now I buried the wrong person' (*News24*, 4 July 2020). Another story, among many, is cited as follows:

> Eastern Cape resident Manono Sozombile is still reeling from the ordeal of reburying his sister-in-law who died of Covid-19 after an undertaker mistakenly delivered the wrong body for burial.
>
> (Citizen, 22 January 2021)

Real stories of these traumatic incidents are confirmed by Chief Mwelo Nonkonyane, the Provincial Chairperson of the Congress of Traditional Leaders of South Africa (CONTRALESA) when he said the following in a live broadcast of the South African Broadcasting Corporation (SABC):

> These things are real and we do have real cases. A person from KwaZulu-Natal was nearly buried in the Eastern Cape, and a body from the Eastern Cape was buried in KwaZulu-Natal and had to be exhumed.
>
> (SABC News, 20 January 2021)

Though Odwa Duru, the owner of the Funeral parlour in Uitenhage says it is critical to enforce Covid-19 regulations, he further says the following about the government rule that one of the reasons the body cannot be viewed is because it comes out already covered with three layers of plastics to prevent the spread of the virus; he further argues:

Quite honestly there is no way. We have to use three-layer plastic. Traditionally, I fully understand the outcry of the people, especially in the Eastern Cape. We do understand. I am Xhosa, I do rituals. I am also appeasing the ancestors. It's not nice, you know, to bury your loved ones, especially the father, mother, you take the body from the mortuary straight to the graveyard without taking the body or coffin to the kraal where we talk to the ancestors.

(SABC News, 20 January 2021)

Several other rituals were banned like the cleansing rituals and the 'putting of stones'; as a result most people claimed that they did not have closure. The government did not take into consideration the nature of African families, and the number of attendees was limited to fifty. For community members not to attend funerals was believed as destroying the basic concept of *ubuntu* that a person is a person because of others. These regulations promoted individualism and a concept of nuclear family which is an import.

On the other hand, these restrictions due to Covid-19 to the practitioners of ATR had some restorative effects. The ban on the night vigils and the morning services was a blessing, as night vigil is a foreign concept to the indigenous faith. Also, the restriction that the body, after being viewed by only nominated elderly family members and then taken straight to the grave, has resulted in bringing back the dignity of funerals. The government reduced the number of days of keeping the body in the morgue as it was required that a person should be buried within three days. This was welcomed by ATR practitioners as they do not see the need to keep the body for a long time in the morgue. In traditional culture a person was buried within three days. As a result, ATR practitioners have now continued with these practices even after Covid-19: there is no night vigil, no morning service involving women, a person is buried within three days, and the service does not take the whole day, but less than two hours. By so doing funeral expenses are cut to a reasonable amount, rather than involving the same expenditure as a wedding. This is the restorative part brought by the pandemic.

References

Dayimani, M. (2020). 'Family Buries Stranger after Covid-19 Body Mix-up'. *News24*. 4 July 2020.

Maliti, S. (2020). 'Double Heartache of Burying Wrong Loved One'. *Daily Dispatch*. 28 July 2020.

Mcetywa, S. A. M. (1991). 'Hermeneutics in the Context of African Traditional Religion with Special Reference to the Mpondo People in Lusikisiki, Flagstaff, and Bizana Areas of Transkei'. M A Thesis. University of Durban-Westville.

Mndende, N. (2020). 'Culture, Spirituality, Religion, and Ritual'. In Richard Hain, Ann Goldman, Adam Rapoport, and Michelle Meiring eds., *Oxford Textbook of Palliative Care for Children*. London: Oxford University Press. 2021.

Omonisi, A. E. (2020). 'The Concept of Death in Africa'. *Pan African Medical Journal 2020* 35 (81).

Sokutu, Brian. (2021). 'Body Mix-up Shocks Family'. *The Citizen*. 22 January 2021.

22

Zarathustra's wisdom: Accepting natural consequences

Jehangir Sarosh

Covid and my religion

When a pandemic such as Covid strikes, the inevitable question is, 'Why does God allow this to happen?' Each religion offers a different perspective on the question, based on its current scientific and prevalent understanding of their scripture. One needs to remember that the scriptures are context-based and yet timeless in their deeper meaning, and it is no different with the Gathas (songs) of Zarathustra. The dialogue in these conversations offers a philosophy of individual responsibility, emphasizing that one cannot abdicate one's responsibility to an authority, not even to the scriptures, and one must be responsible by responding to the need of the moment. The final authority one follows is one's self.

> Hear the best (truth) with your ears and discern by your pure mind; Choose 'the ought' man by man for his/her own self. Before the great trial (comes), wake up to this my counsel.
>
> (Yasna 30.2; in Chatterjee 1967: 87)

This suggests that the ultimate (what some people refer to as God) named Ahura Mazda (Ahura means light and Mazda means Wisdom) in Zoroastrianism or The Light of Wisdom – the inner light energy that illuminates and sustains all there is. In human beings it is the positive and good energy, enabling good thoughts that are formulated into good words and manifested as good actions, while the negative energy operates in darkness due to unconsciousness or ignorance.

Previously, the majority of translations of the Gathas were impressive works of non-Zoroastrian scholars, excellent as they were, but inevitably influenced by their own traditions. For a long period in our history our priests were not educated and they and we had to rely on the translations that were available. In recent years the situation has changed and we are now receiving impressive translations by young Zoroastrians who have studied the Avestan language and the closely related Sanskrit. Many of them are looking deeper into the philosophy of Zarathustra and suggesting that the translation of Ahura should be 'Light' rather than 'Lord'. The Sanskrit word *Asura* has many meanings, including Lord and Light. 'Lord' suggests an authority, and male gender, whereas throughout the Gathas no gender or external authority is implied. 'Light' is preferred, for in virtually all religions, Light is seen as the positive element for it is the light that enlightens. 'The best life is that of who strives for light and shares it with others' (Yasna 43.2).

Furthermore, men and women have been given the ability to connect with Ahura Mazda, the Light of Wisdom, which incorporates knowledge, and through that knowledge one discovers the laws that govern movement and growth. In creation things just happen; however with wisdom and knowledge humans have the ability to facilitate equilibrium. But far too often they have disturbed the equilibrium of nature, as we have experienced from the current ecological climate imbalance which has caused global warming.

Zoroastrianism has been a minority religion and therefore has been heavily influenced by external sources. I believe that the Western conviction that monotheistic philosophy is superior and there has to be only one God has subconsciously put pressure on our community to be seen as modern, 'Western' and not primitive, thereby causing some to claim Zoroastrianism to be monotheistic. Since the majority of Zoroastrians have been educated in Christian schools and colleges, this can seem particularly appealing. The principle of the two primal spirits or energies has often been misunderstood as suggesting that there are two gods in Zoroastrianism. Zarathustra's philosophy is quite clear in suggesting that in the beginning there were two spirits, one positive – Spenta Mainyu – and negative – Angra Mainyu – the two personalities. Often referred to as light and darkness, it clearly recognizes Angra Mainyu (the evil) is an active force. The statements in the Christian Bible, 'Let there be light and there was light' (Gen. 1.3), and 'the darkness comprehended it not' (John 1.5), imply to me that darkness existed before the creation, before the beginning. Pope Paul VI, during a General Audience in 1972, affirmed evil as not merely an absence of something but an active force, a living, spiritual being.

Zarathustra's philosophy suggests that the freedom to choose enables men and women to choose good and thereby to negate the negativity and to overcome ignorance, in communion with Ahura Mazda, the Light of Wisdom. This Light of Wisdom – Ahura Mazda – is the highest source of knowledge, which enables responsible action appropriate to the moment. Thus there is no such being as an external or all-powerful entity in Zarathustra's philosophy. Ahura Mazda is not responsible for what happens in the material creation, such as earthquakes or Covid. They are due to imbalance of the forces prevalent, due to excess or dearth of one aspect of energy that may cause that energy to be where it does not belong, creating disorder. Covid is a virus in the wrong host. Imbalances in nature will continue, and we must learn to recognize what we can change and what is beyond our ability.

Each man and woman has the mind to help him or her connect with the Light of Wisdom and discover the truth, or the cause behind each event, and find a remedy to bring things into balance again. The discovery of the vaccine is an example. Similarly the ecological imbalance can be corrected by identifying the cause of global warming and taking appropriate action. Thus Zarathustra's philosophy confirms the interconnectedness of all there is and the importance of relationships of one with the other. It reminds us of our responsibility to understand and maintain the natural harmony between things, for there is no ultimate authority, no being that has the power to intervene. However negative and destructive, events such as Covid will take place, and individuals and communities have to adjust to the change. One sees that such changes not only affect individuals but families and communities, and Zoroastrians are no exception. Governmental policies of social distancing meant individuals were cut off from the community and media reports made us all aware of the situation, while our isolation caused deep concern for our neighbours and loved ones, resulting in serious mental anguish for some.

Death

The Zoroastrian after-death prayers usually start from the time an individual passes away. All prayers are performed in front of their dear ones, but social distancing laws meant the community had to restrict in-person attendance to the after-death ceremonies. Only two immediate family members could be present and hence not all the traditional rituals were performed. The believers feared the consequences for the departed, leaving some with a feeling of guilt, which may stay with them for a long time. Although the priests were quick in making adaptations and performed all the prayers via Zoom, some elements had to be adjusted in order to limit the risk of spreading Covid. For example, during certain rituals the priests partake in a special ritual handshake, and hold and exchange flowers: all of these were stopped.

The belief in the importance of working in harmony with nature requires minimizing the pollution of the elements of fire, water and air in all stages of life. Thus, according to Zoroastrian tradition, sky burial is the method for disposing of the dead body. Cremation pollutes the air, and burial pollutes the earth. Sky burial disposes of the body in the most ecologically-friendly way. This distinctive Zoroastrian requirement for the disposal of the body forced the community to take measures to overcome the restrictions that were imposed by the government in India. The government's guidelines stated that Covid victims must be cremated, which was contrary to the traditional *Dokhmenashini* system (sky burial), which has been followed for centuries by most Zoroastrians in India. The issue was pursued through the courts and taken all the way to the Supreme Court, which granted the community's right to *Dokhmenashini*. Local communities ensured, wherever possible, that religious ceremonies continued to be performed according to their customs and beliefs, with live-streaming prayers and ceremonies on YouTube, so that the families, loved ones and the community were still able to participate in the departed's ceremony from the safety of their own homes. This was a huge comfort both to the religious leaders and the congregation.

For more pleasurable occasions, the joy of celebrating rites of passage such as weddings, *navjotes* (initiation into the faith community) and other religious festivals had to be postponed or cancelled, as they could not be attended in person. The pandemic has forced communities to continue to review the delivery of services to congregations. Congregations have moved from in-house events only, to hybrid events and live-streaming of prayers and ceremonies for members of the community who cannot attend in person. This has been particularly useful to our community as it is geographically widespread in each country and globally. In many of the congregations the average age is over 60, and older members are therefore classed as vulnerable. However, these changes opened up opportunities for all to participate in festivals, *navjotes*, weddings and funerals. Individuals are by nature social creatures, and less contact is bound to result in isolation and consequent psychological issues, which we hope will be reduced through modern technology, a positive step for all Zarathushti diaspora, offering a greater feeling of belonging to a global community.

Of course, the religious practices will be very different from the way in which ceremonies and festivals have been practised for millennia, Places of worship have traditional design and need to be appropriately equipped with proper live-streaming and audio-visual equipment, while maintaining the necessary ethos for their rituals and prayers. The changes that are taking place have brought home to us the importance of strong commitment to individuals' faith, and for community members to witness the communal prayers and experience the feeling of belonging. By offering webinar facilities, those who cannot attend in person are able to participate in the prayers in the comfort of their homes. Probably the most important change has been the opportunity for each individual to review his or her priorities and evaluate what is needed for a healthy contented life, remembering our interconnectedness with each other and the rest of creation.

The youth were particularly affected by the pandemic, with many of their social activities being cancelled, limiting interaction. However, they were better placed to communicate through the social media and online platforms, where they were able to attend religious classes. Younger children have been deprived of the warmth of friendship of personal contact, and have missed out, both on fun and on learning about our Zoroastrian religion and culture. Although most children could join in the sessions on Zoom it is never the same as meeting with friends in person and sharing each other's stories. Socializing offers the children the opportunity to learn and value the act of sharing. The elderly, being the most vulnerable group, were helped by the young persons in the community, who initiated Care in the Zoroastrian Community (CZC); caring for the elderly and helping those who were completely housebound and had no conventional means of communication. The CZC volunteers made regular phone calls, undertook their daily shopping requirements and offered all kinds of support. A further positive outcome was that it enabled stronger intergenerational connection, enabling new friendships and contacts. The CZC and the rest of the community promoted the UK government vaccination campaign and offered help with taking regular lateral flow tests, while maintaining the relevant safety precautions.

Freedom

There has been much discussion on the freedom to choose whether to wear a mask, but too often freedom and rights have been confused. Rights and freedoms are subject to reasonable limits, which are prescribed by law, and can be justified in a free and democratic society. Yet freedom is not defined by politicians, schools or universities. While they may offer definitions of freedom, it is only when it is curtailed, as by lockdowns, mandatory face masks, social distancing and social exclusion, that we receive some idea of the external freedom we normally enjoy. Such restrictions help us to look deeper within ourselves for our inner freedom to – just be. However, none of these constraints imposed by the pandemic will be permanent, despite Covid's persistence. Let us remind ourselves of the Persian adage, translated and used in several languages: 'This too shall pass.'

References

Chatterji, Jatindra Mohan. (1967). *The Hymns of Atharvan Zarathushtra*. Calcutta: The Parsee Zoroastrian Association. Accessible online at URL: http://www.avesta.org/chatterji/index.html.

Pope Paul VI. (1972). 'Confronting the Devil's Power'. *General Audience*. 15 November 1972. Accessible online at URL: https://www.ewtn.com/catholicism/library/confronting-the-devils-power-8986.

23

Transforming challenges into progress: A Zoroastrian perspective

Koka Karishma

The Zoroastrian Faith is called the *Zarathushti Daena*. *Daena* is a word that combines Conscience and Consciousness. This Path has been given by the prophet Zarathustra who lived in Central Asia several thousand years ago. In the Zoroastrian faith I find messages guided by Ahura Mazda (the Great Wisdom of Creation), for converting challenges into opportunities for good. These guidelines include the principles of sustainable development, entrepreneurship and just action. At the core is spiritual guidance that also impacts the material world, towards creating and sharing true happiness individually and together for the greater good of all. The aim is to make the world a better place through a process called *frashokereti* – which translates as 'to go forward through righteous deeds' and applies collectively and individually.

The prophet Zarathustra is referred to with respect as Asho Zarathustra. The word Asho means pure and righteous. The guidance he has given is preserved in texts called the gāthās – the songs of revelation. In the very first verse here is clear guidance to reach out with outstretched hands and take good righteous action guided by the Good Wisdom of the Mind in order to please the essence or Soul of the Universe (as translated by the Scholar Priest Ervad K. E. Kanga):

Ahyā ỳāsā nemanghā ustānazasto rafadhrahyā maneyush mazdā pourvim spentahyā vispeng shyaothanā vangheush Khraum manangho yā khshnevishāy geushca urvane

I pray at this (moment) in humble adoration with hands uplifted to the invisible (and) bountiful Ahura Mazda, first of all rejoicing all righteous deeds (and) the wisdom of the good mind so that I may please the soul of the universe.

(Yasna 28:1)

This is the essence of responding to crises and removing negativity – in a manner that is based on facts and knowledge such a way that Wisdom is built. As one of the gāthās states, the role of the human being in Zoroastrian belief is to increase the goodness in the world (*Ahura takaesho*) and remove negativity. The belief in Ahura Mazda (the Great Wisdom of Creation) implies that this Energy is in every part of the Universe. Indeed every creation is believed to be guided forward by an essence of this Great Wisdom called the *Fravashi* (which translates as 'to go forward and grow'). It is important to appreciate that the prophet Zarathustra has guided us in his songs of revelation to communicate with Ahura Mazda as one friend to another. This has helped in responding to crises including the Covid pandemic. The principle is utilizing knowledge to guide necessary action.

Cosmic duality is a concept in the Zoroastrian faith that is explained in the texts as dual forces or vectors between which one must choose after listening to the best available knowledge (Yasna Ha 33.3 of the Gāthās). The balance between these two forces is understood to explain the workings of Creation. The positive force is progressive and beneficent, and is referred to as Spenta Mainyu. Indeed a whole gāthā by Zarathustra is named after this concept. This third Gāthā begins with explaining how the six attributes of Ahura Mazda when implemented with this positive force brings about happiness and progress in the world. The opposing vector or negative force is referred to in later Zoroastrian texts as Angra Mainyu and brings about the negative in Creation such as death, calamities and disease, according to some explanations. The role of a Zoroastrian is to increase the positive progressive force through good thought, good words and good deeds (Yasna 47.1).

Scientific analysis has shown that some Covid deaths could have possibly been avoided by taking the vaccines available and participating proactively in mask-wearing, isolation and shielding, as appropriate. This would be explained well by the two principles in the Zoroastrian Faith. The first is Choice with Wisdom in order to make the appropriate decision to discriminate between the two spirits (Spenta Mainyu and Angra Mainyu) (Yasna Ha 33.2 and 33.3). The second is that through good, righteous and benevolent actions one can smite the evil forces (*Druj*) (Yasna Ha 48.1 of the Spenta Mainyu Gāthā). Thus, wearing a mask and isolating help protect others, contributing to saving others from suffering and ill-health. Indeed this has been shown to truly contribute to helping the system combat pandemics like Covid-19. Misinformation is to be avoided through using the intrinsic knowledge together with acquired knowledge (*khratum*). This is key to the principle of building wisdom. Indeed this may have also contributed in some ways to overcoming pandemics.

Being systematic and organized is key to the concept of *ushta* (harmony or happiness), which brings about harmony and happiness. It has been through decades of systematic scientific work on viruses and vaccines that the medical advancements needed to combat Covid-19 were made available within twelve months after the lockdowns started. Equally important, through systematic scientific documentation of the mutations of the virus, further development will be possible to understand the virus and prevent future pandemics. Thus as we can see, the practicalities of implementation of the Zoroastrian precepts can apply to negative circumstances to help overcome challenges and convert them to opportunities for progress.

Listen, reflect, decide

In the Gāthās a verse (Yasna Ha 30.2 and 30.3) guides us to listen, reflect and evaluate with our intellect in each context so that we can turn thoughts to good action. This works at all levels – the individual, the family, entrepreneurial ventures, social development, all the way to *Frashokereti*. which means progressing the world forward through *Asha*: *Fra* means to go forward in fraternity; *Asha* is Righteousness and Purity and Order, and *Kereti* means deeds.

Context-dependent application of information resulted in giving people a choice and a voice leading to equity and empowerment. This principle guided decisions which were taken on the spur of the moment with limited information, but which evolved as more data emerged during the Covid pandemic. As a result we achieved the best outcomes for the community and for individuals, minimizing infections and allowing people to go about their work as safely as possible. An example of this was deciding quite early to stream prayers by Zoom so as to support the community. People prayed together, connected by technology. In the early stages support came from the Zoroastrian Trust Funds of Europe in London, the Californian Zoroastrian Anjuman and the World Zoroastrian Organisation, among others. They opened their sessions to the entire worldwide community. Having such community support is known to benefit the feeling of positivity and the immune system. During the pandemic and even after the lockdown was relaxed, many people continued to participate in prayer sessions online. The advantage of this was to help control the spread of the virus, and it allowed the priests to continue the ritual practices in isolation while supporting the community in the best possible way.

The Zoroastrian principles of Good Thought, Word and Deed were thus put into action. These principles are universal through which we seek to add value for the progress, peace and unity of the world. The Zoroastrian philosophy explains that the two polarities – a progressive mentality (Spenta Mainyu) and a regressive mentality (Angra Mainyu) work simultaneously. Negative occurrences, including disease and death, are the result of the negative. The basis of the Zoroastrian philosophy is to be righteous and good for its own sake at all times without focus on a reward (Ashem Vohu prayer of 12 words). This is also a fine neuro-cognitive principle that brings out the best from the neuro-endocrine system and the immune system in my humble opinion. In the Zoroastrian Prayer (called the Ahunavar which has just 21 words) there is guidance to take good just action guided by the Good Mind, to build good Strength from the Divine and to share what is good with those who need. One thus develops into a caregiver (*vastarem*) who nourishes others. In an important verse in Asho Zarathustra's songs of revelation Zarathustra provides the guidance that 'Happiness comes to those who bring happiness to others'. This spirit of giving is a fundamental pillar of the tenets of Zoroastrianism. However, it does mean that people do not publicize the good work they do. (What the left hand does the right hand does not know.)

Responding during crises

Based on the guidelines mentioned above, during crises such as Covid individuals pull together from all parts of the world's Zoroastrian diaspora to engage in good action and improve the condition of all. Covid was a period of innovation and action in four domains – the social, intellectual, ecological and economic.

Food, care and medical aid were shared free of cost with all who needed it. After death, procedures and care for those left behind were a priority for all Zoroastrian organizations. Priests and community leaders did all that was necessary to the best of their ability to support each and every individual. Response during Covid was a journey from *Asha* (the true ideal righteous plan created with a positive mentality actioned with organization) to *Ushta* (happiness, harmony and progress for all). This involved creating a plan, a path and a progressive environment with a good mind (*vohu manah*). Decisions were taken by organizations based on dialogue and discussion so as to be in accordance with government guidelines.

Collaboration is a key aspect of the Zoroastrian faith. It is guided in the prayers such as the Yenghe Haataam based upon the Gāthic verse Yasna

Ha 51.22. One example of people coming together was an aspect of the International Covid vaccine production, which was supported by many, including the Serum Institute, in collaboration with the University of Oxford. Delivery of the vaccine by Zoroastrians in Iran to people who needed it was achieved by a collaboration between the Zoroastrian Trust Funds of Europe, The World Zoroastrian Organisation Trust Funds and PARZOR (Parsi-Zoroastrian) under the directorship of Dr Shernaz Cama of SOAS (School of Oriental and African Studies, University of London). Education was also supported through online efforts such as an educational network called the Zoroastrian Faculty Network, developed as part of the World Zoroastrian Chamber of Commerce to help students achieve their dreams and gain higher education. Through webinars by people of excellence, students were guided and motivated. It allowed excellent work to lead to growth of knowledge that paves the way to sustainable development.

Imbibing the attributes of the Divine

The Gāthās give us a plan (Verse Yasna Ha 47.1). Ahura Mazda and the attribute Spenta Mainyu (Wisdom and Progressive Understanding) are Ohrmazd's (Ahura Mazda's) principal attributes – with the other characteristics of the Divine Wisdom, including Good Mind (*Vohu Manah*) and Good Order and Purity (*Asha Vahista*), leading to desirable strength or power (*Khshatrem* – which incorporates responsible authority and self-regulation).

When these work with Good Thought, Good Words and Good Actions, together with benevolence and devotion (*Spenta armaity*), they lead to complete holistic welfare or perfection (*Haurvataat*). The combination of imbibing these aspects of the Divine Great Wisdom (Ahura Mazda) leads to harmony and happiness (*ushta*) that lasts through time (*Ameerataat* or immortality) since its foundation is truth and integrity. This is true for the advancement of the group and the individual leading to sustainable development of the organization and society (intellectual, social, economic, ecological) while leading to spiritual advancement. This empowers each one and enables one to empower others, building positivity and emotional resilience with empathy. In Asho Zarathustra, I see a great thought leader who gifts us neuro-cognitive principles helping us adapt to change. This is timeless, time-tested and applies to all domains: entrepreneurship, medicine, ecology, governance, science and engineering, management and business so that the mind (the neural correlate of the brain) and good action can result in building progress through righteousness.

Giving, CSR (Corporate Social Responsibility) and GSR (Green Social Responsibility)

The concept of giving is highlighted in the Gāthās (Yasna Ha 43.1): prosperity, happiness and harmony come to those through whom happiness reaches others. These values, applied for greater good of all, are reflected in CSR and the application of the UN 17 Sustainable Development Goals. As certain industries closed down due to lack of workforce due to Covid, new ideas and enterprises emerged. The education of student priests in India was encouraged by The Incorporated Zoroastrian Charity Funds of Hong Kong, Canton and Macao which funded laptops and other learning support, allowing students to continue their studies.

Sharing knowledge so as to inspire good action was the guiding force in an online programme Ba Humata (with Good Thoughts) founded by Mrs Jerou Panthaki RamMohan and the present author during Covid to help bring the Zoroastrian Community together to take strength from understanding the messages of the faith to take good action in all spheres. Speakers from all over the world were arranged by Meher Amalsad. Priests including Mobed Mehraban Firouzgary and (the late) Mobed Soli P. Dastur provided guidance regarding the prayers. Other lecture series were also instituted including those by Ervad Dr Ramiyar Karanjia and Ervad Darayesh Katrak from Mumbai and Mobed Zarrir Bhandara from California. This kept the emotional, mental and knowledge quotients high, contributing positively to help people emerge from the pandemic. Early in the Covid period the FEZANA (Federation of Zoroastrian Association of North America) talks streamed from the United States brought together students and leaders in different fields. They regularly allowed people to continue their learning. Likewise the North American Mobed Council started an online series to share talks on the prayers that incorporated discussions.

During the COP26 season in October 2021 the Zoroastrian community, like others, sought to bring people of different faiths together to share inspiration and action projects. A webinar series – Progressing Sustainable Together – was set up by the Zoroastrian Trust Funds of Europe (ZTFE) where I was given the opportunity by the ZTFE President Malcolm Deboo and encouraged by Jehangir Sarosh to bring together the essence of the different faiths and those of no faith. Other interfaith work such as that of Jehangir Sarosh through programmes like Conversations across Beliefs and Religions for Peace achieved much good, especially for the youth and school children. Other Zoroastrians like Homi Gandhi and Rohinton Rivetna continued their years of work through programmes at the Parliaments of the World's Religions, which put up an entirely online session. Many Zoroastrians contributed to this interfaith venture. Among the teams were representatives from FEZANA, World Zoroastrian Organization (WZO) Trust Funds and 'The Good Mind – Nurturing Nature' – a Zoroastrian Perspective on Sustainable Development which Mrs Jerou Panthaki RamMohan in London cofounded together with Yazdi Tantra in India and myself. Thus, the three most valuable tenets of Zoroastrianism – Good thoughts, Good Words and Good deeds – proved invaluable during the Covid pandemic.

Reference

Kanga, Ervad Kawasji Edulji (trans.) (1997). *Gatha-Ba-Maani*. in The Religion of Zoroaster. Mumbai: Parsi Panchay. Accessible online at URL: www.zoroaster.com/gatha.htm.

24

Unitarians and global catastrophe: A pandemic, a war and a climate emergency

Feargus O'Connor

What truly reflective, sensitive and caring religious believer can have failed to be profoundly moved and not have felt anguish and sorrow at the millions of deaths and the unprecedented suffering we in our generation have witnessed living through the world's worst health crisis in over a century? At the time of writing we have not only seen at first hand the devastating effects of climate change worldwide but are also witnessing a war causing ever-increasing death and destruction on a massive scale.

The pandemic itself has caused at least 15 million deaths worldwide, over 200,000 in the UK alone. Unknown millions of people of all ages have been infected with the debilitating effects of long Covid, with its symptoms of chronic fatigue, 'brain fog' and shortage of breath: it is estimated that over 2 million in the UK are known to suffer from this distressing and disabling condition. The mental health of many millions more, especially the young, elderly and the clinically vulnerable, has been adversely affected. The crisis has thrown into sharp relief global health and wealth inequalities. This has been particularly stark in the inequitable distribution of clinical care and vaccines worldwide. Is it not scandalous that so many have died needlessly because PPE care equipment and vaccines have not been available to them because of political incompetence, corporate greed and worse?

The pandemic has had an alarming effect on the economies of every country in the world. This has been most devastating for people in the poorest and most economically vulnerable countries in the Third World.

Not only has the education of school children and university students been seriously disrupted but our health systems have been put under unprecedented strain.

Unitarian responses to the pandemic

I can write directly only of my own experience during the pandemic and lockdowns: not only as a minister of a London Unitarian congregation but also in my interfaith capacity as Secretary of the World Congress of Faiths and Chair of the Animal Interfaith Alliance. Sadly, several close ministerial colleagues became ill. I know of a few who contracted long Covid and are still suffering the effects.

In focusing on Unitarian experiences and our religious and humanitarian responses to the pandemic I think it would be illuminating and helpful to refer to the direct involvement of two cherished Unitarian colleagues: Professor Jacqueline Woodman, a consultant obstetrician and gynaecologist, and the Rev. Martin Whitell, London District Minister, who became a volunteer chaplain during the pandemic. Both ministered to and comforted dying Covid-19 patients. Some nights Dr Woodman issued three death certificates, and she herself contracted Covid.

Professor Woodman has told me that the NHS clinical environment changed almost overnight. Elective clinics and surgery stopped as the roll out of PPE and staff testing started. At the height of the first wave of the pandemic, as patient mortality rates soared, specialities like obstetrics implemented the most severe restrictions: women had to give birth with no family members with them: no partners, mothers or sisters, holding their hands and supporting them in what is what she calls the 'most intimate journey' that any mother could make.

The Rev. Martin Whitell advised and visited Unitarian congregations throughout London, gave regular online updates with expert medical advice and he himself volunteered as a chaplain at St Thomas's Hospital, where Florence Nightingale, the daughter of Unitarian parents, walked those wards. Martin tells me that as lockdown impeded many non-clinical services in the hospital and clinical specialists were deployed to Covid-19 care wards and intensive care units the chaplaincy service had urgent demands across the hospital, which had such a reduced workforce.

Not all patients were well enough to be visited and Covid PPE needed to be worn on all the wards. But there were opportunities to converse, offer spiritual care and often pray with infected and recovering patients, those undergoing non-Covid treatment and of course the staff. When major crises arise people are often more open to talk about the important things in life.

Unitarians are emphatically not believers in sacramental and ritualistic religion and so the lack of in-person services presents no theological difficulties. Throughout the pandemic, particularly during the periods of lockdown, wearing a mask and keeping the required social distancing, I paid regular pastoral visits, sent weekly in-touch emails with the texts of services and kept in regular contact with congregational members by telephone. From April 2020 we began, and still continue to offer, Zoom services and other online spiritual activities. After the lockdowns ended we decided to hold in-person, hybrid and Zoom services as many individuals, some from as far afield as the Netherlands and the United States as well as from various parts of the UK, requested continuing Zoom services as they appreciated these so much. Interestingly, the same pattern has occurred with our EC meetings of the World Congress of Faiths, Animal Interfaith Alliance, London District Unitarian Council and the editorial board of *The Inquirer*, our national Unitarian paper. In each case we continue to have our meetings on Zoom and so save money and cut down on unnecessary travel.

Thanks to scrupulously observing all lockdown measures and, upon re-opening our chapel for in-person services and other congregational activities, by dint of following rigorous health and safety precautions, including social distancing, thorough hygienic routines and the wearing of face coverings, only two members of my Golders Green congregation actually contracted Covid-19. Fortunately in each case it was a mild dose of the Omicron variant.

Religious and moral reflections on the lessons learned

Writing as an individual Unitarian minister and reflecting only my own views and conclusions, I feel that this pandemic has brought out of people the best and the worst: the spirit of empathy and kindness on the part of so many millions of caring fellow citizens but also selfishness, callousness, individual and corporate greed. We have witnessed reckless disregard for others on the part of irresponsible and menacing 'anti-vaxxer' crowds and populist demagogues in the United States, Brazil and elsewhere who encouraged their followers to ignore the relevant scientific evidence and so put many millions of lives at risk.

In the spirit of the Charter for Compassion, which was adopted by UK Unitarians following a Unitarian General Assembly resolution in 2011, and of another General Assembly resolution (2012), which I also moved, honouring our co-religionist Clara Barton, the founder of the American Red Cross, and instituting a special appeal by the British Red Cross to support its various lifesaving emergency appeals, UK Unitarians have raised over £200,000 for such Red Cross crisis appeals.

In April 2020 I drafted an emergency national appeal calling on Unitarians throughout Britain to contribute to both the British Red Cross Global and its UK Coronavirus Crisis Appeals. I am pleased that many thousands of pounds were donated, and that this was the single most significant humanitarian response by Unitarians nationwide. We responded with practical compassion by sending medical and other humanitarian aid to alleviate the suffering of millions of people in Yemen, Syria, Gaza and other Palestinian Territories, Somalia, Afghanistan and Rohingya refugee camps in Bangladesh, where we witnessed a surge in coronavirus infections devastating those countries and spiralling out of control. The death toll was steadily increasing, hospital beds were full and there was a desperate need to provide essential medical supplies and treatment facilities for these vulnerable communities, many the victims of war and destitute refugees whose lives remained, and remain, in acute and immediate danger.

The Charter for Compassion, which Unitarians embrace, embodies the Golden Rule, which is at the heart of the great world religions and ethical philosophies, East and West, and that spirit of empathy and compassion which, as Dr Albert Schweitzer and other religious humanitarians have proclaimed, is surely the hallmark of all authentic and truly engaged religion? That spirit of empathy impelled Unitarians, like so many others, to act to help save precious human lives during the pandemic by supporting not only Red Cross Global and UK Coronavirus Appeals but also those launched for the suffering people of Yemen, Afghanistan and Syria. We have since raised large sums for victims of the war in Ukraine. This humanitarian response to aid the victims of the pandemic and war was our most significant act of practical compassion expressing our core religious and ethical ideals.

Nowhere has this moral impulse been better expressed than in these proclamations by two of the world's great religions of the illimitable worth, innate dignity and unique destiny of every human soul.

Whoever destroys a soul, it is considered as if he destroyed an entire world. And whoever saves a life, it is considered as if he saved an entire world.

(*Jerusalem Talmud*, Sanhedrin 4:1: 22a)

Whosoever killeth a human being … it shall be as if he had killed all mankind, and whosoever saveth the life of one, it shall be as if he had saved the life of all mankind.

(*The Qur'an*, Surah Al-Ma'idah, verse 5:32, Pickthall translation)

As I write we are confronting another global disaster. The most dangerous and destructive war since 1945 is raging in Ukraine. We face the worst political crisis since the Second World War and the tragedies of the Holocaust, Hiroshima and Nagasaki.

I recall words of the Quaker MP and peace advocate John Bright, who in a speech delivered to a conference of the Peace Society in Edinburgh in October 1853, just before the outbreak of the Crimean War, took a determined moral stand against another war involving Russia and one in which Leo Tolstoy served and first witnessed what Martin Luther King called the 'madness of war'. In that speech Bright condemned *war itself* as the 'combination and concentration of all the horrors, atrocities, crimes, and sufferings of which human nature on this globe is capable'. He warned of the perils of a 'bloody, unjust, and unnecessary war ... perils into which unthinking men – men who do not intend to fight themselves – are willing to drag or to hurry this country. I am amazed how they can trifle with interests so vast and consequences so much beyond their calculation.'

Unlike the Covid-19 unseen killer we combat in this pandemic, war is a calculated act: a grave sin against God and crime against humanity caused by human evil, vanity and criminal folly. Those who pour billions of dollars of arms to perpetuate this disastrous war with all its resultant deaths and destruction, global food shortages and other often unforeseen disasters, coming as they do amidst the sufferings of billions of people still just recovering from that pandemic, are surely guilty of the gravest of sins?

Tolstoy, Gandhi, Schweitzer, Martin Luther King, Thich Nhat Hanh, Desmond Tutu and other religious apostles of non-violence would surely have agreed. As Rabbi Abraham Joshua Heschel wrote, the 'choice is to love together or perish together'. Words echoed by his friend Martin Luther King, who said that the choice was 'no longer between violence and non-violence' but rather between 'non-violence and non-existence'.

This hard-won understanding of the interconnectedness of all living beings and of the moral imperative to strive for the common good surely constitutes the vital lesson which this global pandemic, the war in Ukraine and the moral and religious duty to take determined action in this climate emergency all teach us? But *will* we act in time?

One Unitarian view on whether there can be a convincing theodicy

But do such sufferings not raise profound religious questions, none more urgent than whether we can ever find a truly convincing and coherent theodicy? As a Unitarian Universalist who does not believe in any form of 'revealed' religion and so has conscience, reason and empathy for the sufferings of all fellow beings as my sole guides, I find, both in my heart and head, the dogmas of all creedal religions unconvincing. So I value doubt and scepticism all the more.

Witnessing as we do so many millions of deaths in this worldwide pandemic, the devastating consequences of climate change and the war now raging in Ukraine, with all the mass slaughter of innocents, maimed bodies, widespread destruction and despair of those who survive and mourn, surely only the most dogmatic and uncritical believers can have failed to examine the essentials of their religious faith? Have they themselves not agonized over such heartfelt questions as 'Why is such suffering tolerated by a supposedly just and loving Divine dispensation?' and 'Can we really believe in an interventionist God?'

For many philosophers, and even some more sceptical and incisive theologians, does not the prevalence of widespread suffering caused by pandemics and wars provide very strong evidence that serves to undermine the essential beliefs and presuppositions of Classical Theism? 'Epicurus's old questions are yet unanswered. Is he willing to prevent evil, but not able? Then is he impotent. Is he able, but not willing? Then is he malevolent. Is he both able and willing? Whence then is evil?' (Hume [1779] 1993: 100). In these penetrating words of Epicurus, quoted by the Humean sceptic Philo in Part 10 of David Hume's posthumously published philosophic time bomb *Dialogues Concerning Natural Religion* (1779), Hume encapsulates the essential 'Problem of Evil', surely one of the most devastating arguments in the arsenal of atheistic opponents of established 'revealed' religions?

For any theodicy to be really convincing, as the Process philosopher of religion David Ray Griffin has argued, it must be rationally persuasive and plausible as well as offer logically possible propositions. Those of dogmatic Christian apologists like Richard Swinburne and Alvin Plantinga, to my mind, do not pass that test. Though I am more sympathetic to John Hick's well-worked-out liberal Christian theodicy of 'soul making' in opposition to the traditional Augustinian one I find so revolting to both reason and conscience, I think the main weakness of Hick's is its adherence to what Griffin himself has called the 'omnipotence fallacy': that is the view that God is 'limitlessly powerful'.

Though we may not be personally convinced by all the arguments of the Process philosophers and theologians in the honourable tradition of Alfred North Whitehead we may agree with that philosopher's perceptive observation that many orthodox apologists have had a marked tendency to 'pay God metaphysical compliments' as if 'He' were an Eastern potentate or absolute monarch craving flattery. These sycophantic compliments, as Hume charged, 'savour more of panegyric than of philosophy'.

This tentative Process theism, though it is not of course susceptible to absolute philosophic proof, seems to accord with, or at least it does not conflict with, the facts of the cosmos as we presently apprehend them. In particular, its open-minded attitude to the survival of our individual personalities and consciousness after death may help form the basis of a bold theodicy which can look beyond our individual short lifespans and give us grounds for hope that our present sufferings, injustices and inequalities are not the end of the story.

Like Demea, a character in Hume's *Dialogues,* we may embrace 'larger views' and look to a future life and a hope for Cosmic justice beyond the absurd injustices of our present brief existence on this planet. May we not indeed hope that death will not cancel and expunge all our individual minds and unique personalities and that we may be given redress for all the seemingly unjust sufferings and anguish we have to endure here on earth? Like countless millions of believers in diverse religious traditions may we not still hope that we shall look back upon the pains and struggles of this present life and ultimately understand their full significance in whatever life there is hereafter? Is this a reasonable or is it a vain hope?

References

Alicia. (2018). 'We Have It within Us to Save a Life'. Accessible online at URL: http://kineticmotions.ca/save-life.

Hume, David (ed. J. C. A. Gaskin) ([1779] 1993). *Dialogues Concerning Natural Religion.* Oxford: Oxford University Press.

Pickthall, Marmaduke (trans.) (1977). *The Meaning of the Glorious Coran.* Beirut: Dar Al-Kitab Allubnani.

25

Unitarian Universalists face Covid: Challenges, surprises and new pathways

Jay Atkinson

Unitarian and Universalist churches exist on six continents, ranging across social and economic circumstances far too diverse to permit any synoptic coverage. My colleague, Feargus O'Connor, addresses the situation in the UK. Here I limit my attention to Unitarian Universalist churches in the United States, in whose ministry I have served since 1979.

Theology, anthropology and ethics

Because Unitarian Universalism (UU) is a theologically diverse movement in the United States, no single religious interpretation of the Covid phenomenon is possible. Broadly speaking, however, we can say that almost all laity and clergy in our UU congregations share views that lean strongly in humanistic and naturalistic directions and away from any supernatural explanations of events, good or bad. We are not at all inclined, as are some more conservative churches, to interpret natural disasters as the punishing actions of a divine ruler.

Views of 'God' span a wide spectrum among our members. Some have no use for the word at all. Theists among us conceive God in a variety of ways, but nearly all would understand divine power as being entirely consistent with the reality of human freedom, moral agency and the inherent worth and dignity of human life. Many of us embrace open and relational theologies (in either Christian or non-Christian forms) that emphasize *Love* as the primary divine attribute and interpret God's power in the world as a purely spiritual force that continually encourages us in the direction of goodness. In this view, God does not and cannot intervene physically or coercively to initiate, control or prevent destructive events in the world. It is we who by our freely chosen response to the persuasion of God's love may answer the call to work for a human society of peace, justice and cooperation for our collective safety and the common good.

Unitarian Universalists generally have a keen interest in living and working for the common good of their local communities as well as Earth's global human family and the physical health of the planet itself. This comes, in part, from a long history, going back to the sixteenth century, of understanding the religious life as fundamentally ethical in character. Very early in the Reformation, Unitarians and their forebears moved away from typical Protestant understandings of justification by grace through faith, and especially from the Reformed doctrine of predestination, and towards a view of salvation based on following the life of Jesus as a model for righteous living. Human beings were understood as free agents guided by conscience and the Hebrew prophetic tradition of justice and living in caring relationship with others as the proper expression of obedience to God.

The idealism of this view must reckon with the reality that human beings often use their freedom for venal and self-serving ends. The Covid pandemic brought such behaviour to light. In China it seems that medical personnel were slow or even dishonest in reporting the extent and severity of the Covid threat. In the United States medical data were likewise manipulated or concealed for political gain. Most Unitarian Universalists understand that, even in the presence of a universal or divine lure towards the good, our world can be a dangerous arena of ill fortune and natural disaster. While neither we – nor God! – can do much to prevent the *incidence* of such adversities, we can and should work with one another to mitigate their effects and relieve the suffering that may follow them. When we do this work, we become, in the words of Teresa of Ávila, 'the hands and feet of God'. Atheists among us might express human responsibility in more worldly terms, but a shared commitment to the common good still prevails across the spectrum of UU thinking and action.

The natural world presents us with many challenges and dangers, and we must collaborate with one another in using our gifts of reason and scientific inquiry to understand their workings and learn how to protect ourselves from their ravages. On this basis we welcome the scientific understanding of nature as an essential source of knowledge for our shared work of promoting human health and well-being in mutuality with the natural processes of our planetary environment.

Congregational life and worship

With the onset of Covid-19, our congregations in the United States were quick to suspend all gathering in person for worship. A majority, with surprising agility, were able to reconceive their programmes of communal worship, education, and social fellowship through video links and electronic applications like *Zoom*. For smaller congregations the learning curve was steeper and more challenging, but after a few bumps, most of them developed the requisite skill for maintaining basic congregational programmes through video communication.

UU churches, though not primarily Christian in theology, still follow mostly Protestant patterns of communal worship. To a significant extent this means that preaching and the spoken word continue to occupy a central role in UU worship. The downside of this has been that some of the visual elements of worship have often not been given the attention they deserve. The advent of Covid brought this need into newly sharpened focus. Suddenly taken from us were the most familiar visual accompaniments of communal worship – windows telling stories in stained glass images or opening transparently on to living natural expanses of tree and flower, flames flickering up from candle or chalice as leaping reminders of hope, of truth, of human warmth and the reassuring presence of friends sitting beside us, offering us their smiling faces, the familiar clasp of hands or an open-armed hug. We have had to supplant the spiritual and emotional force of these elements of worship by weaker and sometimes more awkward alternatives.

One of the most frequent processional hymns used in formal UU gatherings begins:

Rank by rank again we stand, from the four winds gathered hither, Loud the hallowed walls demand, whence we come and how, and whither.

(Unitarian Universalist Association 1993, no. 358)

When Covid made physical gathering no longer possible and 'hallowed walls' became only a figurative reference, there was a serious loss of the solace that comes from familiarity of space itself. Ideally in our tradition (as in many others, of course), communal worship is an activity – indeed, a spiritual practice – in which those assembled feel safe in opening themselves vulnerably to grow, to change, to receive new insight, to take new resolve, maybe even to embrace a new vision. That feeling of safety comes, in part, from being surrounded by familiar walls and sitting in the presence of familiar friends.

Some of our largest churches were quickly able to continue conducting communal worship from their usual chancels and sanctuaries, even without the presence of any congregants in the pews. Many more ministers, however, began preaching and leading worship in a seated posture from home offices, living rooms or makeshift 'studios'. Musicians appeared at their home pianos or just as 'singing heads'. It was all very strange and required new ways of feeling worshipful.

As a retired minister striving to participate in congregational life remotely from my computer screen, I was immediately drawn to Zooming into worship with those congregations whose ministers, worship associates and musicians were able to speak, sing and play from the familiar formal settings of pulpit and chancel. The visual impact was inspiriting for me in ways that a casually dressed minister speaking and preaching from an informal space was not.

Yet UU congregational life is not all about formal worship. We also value opportunities for social interaction in coffee hours after Sunday worship, for growth in knowledge and understanding through classes that offer study and discussion of theological, historical, ethical and political topics, and for building deeper and more trustful interpersonal relationships through participation in smaller and more intimate circles in which sharing of emotionally laden feelings and experiences can be practised. While the use of Zoom technology was initially seen as a forced and unhappy choice, the surprising result has been that many aspects of these experiences have proved to be *enhanced* by the new format. Church members whose shyness previously kept them standing aside during the coffee hour have found that the video technology of 'breakout rooms' has invited them to enter more comfortably into meaningful conversation and to make new and deeper friendships. The same is true for more welcoming and equitable participation in adult education classes and small-group ministries.

The replacement of in-person worship with video technology has had mixed effects. Some congregations have suffered severe cutbacks in financial support, while others, surprisingly, have seen many of their members rise to the occasion with stronger levels of giving. Elders who have been shut out from worship for lack of physical mobility or convenient transportation have found themselves newly able to feel like full participants in their own churches. Others who have moved away to new homes, sometimes quite far away, and who in earlier times would have transferred their church membership to the new location, have instead, with new flexibility, maintained their existing congregational allegiance and financial support despite the distance. In addition, the option of joining into communal worship remotely has actually resulted in membership growth for some congregations, not only from people who live locally but also from some who have discovered a congregation by internet connection from quite far away, across the country or even across an ocean. It is truly a new era, and the longer-term impact of these varied patterns remains to be seen as we move out of the most acute phases of the Covid pandemic.

The work of the clergy

The stresses resulting from Covid have fallen particularly hard upon clergy. Parish ministry is often experienced as stressful, even under ordinary circumstances. Many of our clergy report being overwhelmed by unprecedented levels of exhaustion. Some have negotiated reduced levels of service with their congregations, and a few have felt compelled to resign their positions just to take a deep breath and bring their lives and health back into balance.

At the same time, workloads have been eased by new forms of congregational cooperation. In many instances two or more of our ministers have agreed to share their sermons or even their entire hours of worship with one another, preaching by video to multiple congregations simultaneously or by delayed replay, thus reducing the number of sermons needing to be prepared by any one minister, beneficially exposing congregations to a wider variety of preaching perspectives and worship styles, and promoting improved levels of mutual congregational acquaintance and interdependence.

Pastoral conversations, typically taking place in the home of a parishioner or in the privacy of the minister's office, have shifted rather easily into the mode of private video conferencing. While some of the intimacy of physical presence is lost, the ability to reach out without the need to travel and to be available at more flexible times of day has facilitated the pastoral aspect of our ministry.

Other positive surprises

Unitarian Universalists have long been committed to environmental justice and to caring for our planet. The carbon footprint of air travel has been a particular point of frustration even as we continued to believe, in pre-pandemic times, that in-person meetings of committees were necessary for the efficient functioning of our UU movement at the national level.

We were wrong. With reduced travel imposed on us during the pandemic, nearly all nationwide conferences and committee meetings had to be conducted via Zoom, and many participants were pleasantly surprised to discover how well this worked out, especially how it facilitated patterns and styles of interaction, through small-group breakout rooms, that would not have happened with usual in-person gatherings.

Emerging and lasting impacts

With the advent of effective Covid vaccines, our UU congregations have cautiously begun to welcome members back into their physical sanctuaries. But not all are vaccinated, some out of distrust of the vaccine and the science behind it, some because of auto-immune and other pre-existing medical conditions for whom vaccination constitutes serious dangers. Navigating tensions between ideals of fairness, inclusion and safety has posed difficult questions for our congregations' clergy and lay leaders, with no single pathway of resolution. Excluding the unvaccinated, for whatever reason, runs counter to our commitment to radical inclusiveness. But the safety of our children must, at the same time, be a high priority. Our best hope is for the day – may it be soon! – when we can move beyond 'either/or' and embrace everyone in the spirit of 'both/and'.

Illness, natural disaster and loss are experiences that often provoke crises of faith, moving people to question previously comfortable and comforting worldviews and to ask for reasons why such events happen. While most UUs, as described in the opening section of this chapter, have seemed satisfied with the understanding that such things are random and not the result of malevolent or punishing forces, some may nonetheless find themselves asking deeper questions about life's meaning and vicissitudes. One prominent UU minister reported, several months into the pandemic, that 'I have never seen the people I serve hungrier for theological thought. These days, ministers are obviously not just managers or CEOs, but public theologians who are imperfectly, authentically making meaning in front of people – all while inviting them to do the same' (Nancy McDonald Ladd; quoted in Eaton 2021).

As we emerge cautiously from the most acute phases of the Covid pandemic (or so it seems at the moment of this writing – June 2022), it is too soon to discern all the lessons of these past two years, but a few things are already clear. More and more congregations have begun 'multi-platform' worship, with in-person gathering that is simultaneously available remotely to people 'zooming' in to listen and participate. Preaching to more than a thousand Unitarian Universalists gathered at our annual General Assembly in June 2022, one of our ministers wondered aloud what it means to 'do and be church' in a looming post-pandemic reality: 'What if ownership and maintenance of a church building may actually be an obstacle to "doing church" in the future?' she asked.

At the level of our national organization, many staff people are now scattered around the country working remotely without the need for a desk or office cubicle in our headquarters building. In a strange irony, this pandemic has opened new possibilities and modes of common work. The transformation is still in process, and we are caught up in the flow of its uncertain impacts. Its currents are carrying us forward into a new era whose contours are only dimly visible at present.

References

Eaton, Joshua. (2021). 'Pandemic Reckoning'. *UUWorld*. Spring, 1 May. Accessible online at URL: www.uuworld.org/articles/pandemic-reckoning.

Unitarian Universalist Association. (1993). *Singing the Living Tradition*. Boston: Beacon Press.

26

When 'No resident will say: "I am sick"': The global religious response of Jehovah's Witnesses to the Covid-19 pandemic

Jolene Chu

For Jehovah's Witnesses the holiest day of the year is the Memorial of the death of Jesus Christ, held annually on Nisan 14, according to the biblical lunar calendar. Congregants and their guests usually gather in Kingdom Halls for a Bible lecture and simple commemoration, during which red wine and unleavened bread are passed to attendees as symbols of Jesus's sacrifice. In 2019, nearly twenty-one million attended the Memorial.

In 2020, the Memorial fell on April 7, not quite one month after the World Health Organization declared Covid-19 a global pandemic. By the time of the Memorial, the Witnesses had already suspended in-person religious activities worldwide: congregations were holding virtual worship services, and the Witnesses' signature door-to-door ministry had been replaced by outreach via telephone, letter and videoconferencing, as permitted by local law. Over seventeen million viewed the 2020 Memorial via live-streamed or pre-recorded commemorations. Though the recorded attendance was considerably less than the previous year, a wide, unnumbered audience could access the programme via video stream, radio and television broadcasts hastily arranged days before the Memorial.

Jehovah's Witnesses are an international Christian community numbering 8.7 million in 239 lands. The ecclesiastical Governing Body of Jehovah's Witnesses provides religious direction and guidance to Jehovah's Witnesses worldwide. The congregational activity of Jehovah's Witnesses is coordinated by branch offices under the direction of the Witnesses' world headquarters in New York.

The development of Covid measures related to the Witnesses' religious activities has been supervised from world headquarters. Since pandemic conditions varied from region to region, some measures were applied globally and others locally, in harmony with governmental regulations. Global directives included the cancellation of live events, including the large annual conventions scheduled to begin in May 2020, and their replacement with a virtual programme. The convention programme's 114 audio-video segments had already been produced, but about forty lectures – typically delivered live by local speakers worldwide – had to be recorded in English and then translated and dubbed in more than 500 languages. This mammoth effort began as soon as the cancellation was announced in March. It was accomplished, initially in 400 languages, with the opening programme posted to the Witnesses' official website, jw.org, on 6 July 2020.

Activities such as ministerial and organizational training courses, pastoral visitation, international delegations and other gatherings transitioned to virtual formats. Construction projects at branch facilities and meeting places were suspended. Safe and creative solutions had to be found to conduct other collaborative work, such as the preparation, translation, and production of literature, audio recordings and video programming.

The Governing Body articulated three guidelines drawn from Bible principles on which pandemic measures would be determined:

1   Follow governmental regulations; respect public health recommendations, based on Rom. 13.1: 'Let every person be in subjection to the superior [secular] authorities.'

2   Adopt health precautions that place a high value on life, based on Eccl. 7.12: 'Wisdom preserves the life of its owner.'

3   Avoid casual attitudes and premature resumption of activities, based on Prov. 22.3: 'The shrewd one sees the danger and conceals himself' (JW 2020).

These principles were aligned with core teachings of the Witnesses' faith to determine how they would carry on their worship during the pandemic.

The name Jehovah's Witnesses embodies the primary role that believers assume upon baptism into the faith. This designation is drawn from the

Bible book of Isaiah, where God, Jehovah, says to the nation of Israel: 'You are my witnesses.' The Israelites would live by God's law given through Moses, and their continued existence would testify that God had fulfilled his promises in their behalf (Isa. 43.10, 12). Witnesses today see themselves as serving in a similar role, living by divine standards and bearing witness about Jehovah, an activity mandated by Jesus and practised by the early Christians (Acts 1.8; 20.20).

Consistent with their belief that Christ (Messiah) will one day rule over a paradise earth without humanly constructed borders and divisions, Witnesses attempt to reach all people with 'this good news of the Kingdom' (Mt. 24.14). Their outreach includes distributing free Bible literature and, more recently, digital material accessible on their official website. Consistent with the Witnesses' borderless worldview, jw.org has content in over 1,050 languages, including more than 100 sign languages. Being the most widely translated website in the world, jw.org has enabled Witnesses to continue their Bible education work using this safe method to share a message of hope in the face of worldwide distress.

Jehovah's Witnesses believe that the world is experiencing the 'last days' of human rulership, as the Bible foretold (Mt. 24; Mk 13; Lk. 21; 2 Tim. 3; Rev. 6.1-8). The Witnesses expect this period – marked by war, lawlessness, famine, pestilence and fear – to culminate in the fulfilment of the Lord's prayer: 'Let your will take place, as in heaven, also on earth' (Mt. 6.10, NWT).

While the Witnesses view pandemics as evidence of the 'last days', they do not attribute special prophetic significance to the Covid pandemic, nor do they view pandemics and other natural disasters as divine punishment. As Witnesses observe or experience such tragic happenings, they believe they have reason for optimism that divine relief is close at hand. Still, embracing this future hope does not induce fatalistic apathy towards present suffering. Despite their own pandemic-related challenges, Witnesses in 2020 and 2021 devoted over three billion hours to their ministry. In normal times, Witnesses who engage in this self-supported charitable work personally fund the fuel or public transportation that takes them to neighbourhoods across the globe. During the pandemic, they instead made phone calls and bought postage to send millions of letters, many of them carefully composed and handwritten, to console their neighbours.

The Witnesses' response to Covid has also been guided by biblical doctrine regarding obedience to secular law. They believe that Christ's command to 'render Caesar's things to Caesar' requires Christians to obey civil authority unless it conflicts with divine law (Mt. 22.21; Rom. 13.1-7). So, while the Witnesses continue to obey God by their worship and witnessing, they also observe Covid-related government mandates, including science-based public health directives. Where warranted for health and safety, congregations observe more stringent health measures than required by law.

Beginning in late February 2020, official communications to congregations strongly encouraged basic safety measures, such as regular handwashing and mask-wearing. Some branches distributed sanitizing kits to Witness homes, and all branch and headquarters staff were required to wear masks and practise physical distancing.

The organization reiterated its long-held position that, as with other medications, the choice to be vaccinated is a personal matter. The Governing Body explicitly stated their official view that 'there is no religious objection to vaccination' (JW n.d.). Over 99 per cent of the headquarters staff chose to be vaccinated, with similar rates in branch offices worldwide.

Maintaining congregation life

Congregation meetings are a crucial means of spiritual instruction and social support for the community. The organization took steps to ensure accessibility to meetings, such as by negotiating favourable rates for Zoom accounts for congregation use worldwide. By June 2020, over 65,000 congregations in 170 countries were using Zoom for virtual meetings. In economically disadvantaged areas, spiritual programmes were and continue to be brought to homes by JW Satellite, a free television broadcast service, and by purchased television and radio airtime. Thus, the 2020 Memorial was broadcast in at least twenty-four languages and reached about 407,000 Witnesses in sub-Saharan Africa, along with an undetermined number of other viewers. Where internet connectivity is limited or expensive, a low-cost, custom-designed router and digital storage device called JW Box has allowed for wireless transfers of pre-recorded programmes to electronic devices.

The Witnesses' meetings are highly participatory, with question-and-answer segments, model teaching demonstrations and whole-congregation singing. The transition to virtual meetings required coordinated efforts to help connect elderly ones and others unfamiliar with videoconferencing tools. A 2022 study of Jehovah's Witnesses in Spain compared perceptions of in-person versus virtual meetings with respect to transcendent experience, intellectual learning and teaching, and social interaction. The study found that virtual attendees still felt strongly connected to God during prayers but less so when singing songs. When delivering talks, speakers evaluated the in-person and virtual settings comparably, although audience reaction on screen could not be so easily discerned. In-person social interaction was judged greatly superior to on-screen interchanges. Virtual attendees reported a strong perception of being taught by God, evidence that 'Jehovah's Witnesses continue to consider meetings as a way of listening to their God no matter what the medium' (Torres-Pruñonosa, Plaza-Navas and Brown 2022).

The Witnesses' public ministry is core to their religious identity. Baptized and unbaptized Witnesses who engage in the ministry are called 'publishers' because they publicize the 'good news of the Kingdom' – by 'preaching' to the general public and by 'teaching' those who welcome further engagement on biblical topics. Witnesses individually decide how much time they spend, but they often preach and teach together for mutual exchange and encouragement.

Virtually overnight, the sight of Witnesses at doorsteps and with public literature displays pivoted to remote preaching and teaching. Using public directories where permitted by law, they wrote letters and made brief telephone calls that often included a Bible verse and an invitation to visit jw.org for its free content on topics such as coping with isolation and pandemic fatigue, remote learning, avoiding misinformation and conspiracy theories, help for victims of domestic abuse and controlling alcohol consumption.

During the pandemic, Witnesses have conducted free, one-on-one Bible study courses with millions of people by video or telephone. The course typically takes months or even a year or more to complete. Subsequently, some Bible students have decided to be baptized as Jehovah's Witnesses, and that was without ever having set foot in a Kingdom Hall. They, in turn, began sharing in preaching and teaching, the work that Witnesses consider integral to their worship and a tangible expression of their love for God and neighbour (Mt. 22.37-39).

Global pandemic measures

There are no salaried positions at any level of the organization, including its headquarters and branch offices, where resident workers receive only a modest stipend. Likewise, elders in local congregations are not employees, nor do they receive any remuneration for their services, all functions being supported by voluntary donations.

Each congregation is overseen by a body of elders, spiritually qualified men who lead the congregants in worship and extend pastoral care. In times of crisis, elders endeavour to maintain contact with all congregants, keeping them informed and ascertaining their situations and needs. Besides the mutual help offered spontaneously by individual believers, local elders collaborate with branch offices in providing spiritual and practical support (Domaradzki 2022). In turn, branch offices provide the world headquarters with real-time reports of conditions on the ground to help formulate and implement disaster preparedness and response plans. This organizational infrastructure, from the local to global level, enables timely two-way information-gathering and dissemination of guidance and practical assistance.

Branch offices appoint Disaster Relief Committees (DRCs) to coordinate trained rapid-response teams. The DRCs assess the needs, distribute relief supplies, organize evacuations, repair or replace damaged homes and perform other vital services with funds allocated by the organization. The organization's disaster preparedness arrangements are described in the video *2019 Coordinators' Committee Report – Supporting Our Brothers When Disasters Strike*. During the pandemic, over 950 DRCs mobilized thousands of volunteer relief workers worldwide to supply food, medical supplies and sanitizing kits to vulnerable Witness households. In some locations, DRCs assisted in locating open hospital beds and oxygen supplies, and Witness medical professionals volunteered to provide telemedicine assistance. By January 2021, over twenty-five million dollars (US) in donations had been allocated to DRCs for Covid relief.

Since the pandemic caused the suspension of construction and maintenance projects, additional personnel became available for Covid relief work. DRCs also continued handling other disasters. In one 12-month period in 2020–1, DRCs responded to over 200 disasters, including floods, hurricanes, volcanic eruptions and wildfires.

The jw.org website played a crucial role in fostering a sense of unity and calm in the Witness community. Beginning on 18 March 2020, Governing Body members regularly addressed Witnesses worldwide with video updates on pandemic-related matters. The updates, posted to jw.org in hundreds of languages, offer spiritual advice, consolation for those suffering loss, international reports and interviews of ordinary Witnesses about coping with lockdown, illness, unemployment, depression, anxiety, civil unrest and other difficulties. Witnesses were encouraged to inform congregation elders of their needs and not to hesitate to accept help. Two programmes focused on how parents may help their children deal with stress.

Governing Body members urged patience and continued vigilance, cautioning against being influenced by conspiracy theories and popular resistance to public health measures. Underscoring the seriousness of this counsel were announcements of the rate of hospitalization and death among Witnesses. The death toll stood at 26,813 as of January 2022. Many of those who succumbed lived in areas with high infection rates and limited access to vaccines. Others reportedly had underlying health conditions. While acknowledging that vaccination remains a matter of personal choice, Witnesses were encouraged to consider the evidence that vaccines had proven effective in lowering rates of hospitalization and death.

In early 2022, with the increase of vaccination rates and treatment options and the drop in infections, conditions seemed favourable to consider a return to in-person activities.

Resumption of activities

On 1 April 2022, two weeks before the annual Memorial commemoration, local congregations began holding hybrid (combined in-person and virtual) meetings, including the Memorial, where local conditions permitted. Mask-wearing has been strongly recommended. As occurred at the outset of the pandemic, some 120,000 congregations scrambled to prepare, this time to open Kingdom Halls and equip them to accommodate virtual participants. Those with limiting circumstances will now benefit from the permanent option of hybrid meetings. Congregations may also face fewer disruptions due to public health threats and other unforeseen conditions.

On 31 May 2022, the Governing Body announced the end of the historic suspension of the Witnesses' in-person ministry. Effective 1 June 2022, Witnesses resumed the public ministry, with the exception of door-to-door visitation. Almost immediately, Witnesses wearing face masks appeared with mobile literature carts on streets and in public parks. The door-to-door ministry resumed on 1 September 2022.

The pandemic's full effect on Jehovah's Witnesses and their ministry work has yet to be quantified. Biblically based guidance, an organized infrastructure and a tradition of volunteerism have enabled Witnesses to adapt during the pandemic. While physical distancing and virtual interaction could have weakened bonds of fellowship, uninterrupted worship services, community outreach and mutual help served to strengthen them. For many Witnesses, the pandemic has brought into clearer focus biblical prophecies concerning the 'last days' and given fresh meaning to their hopeful message that one day, under God's Kingdom, 'No resident will say: "I am sick"' (Isa. 33.24).

References

Domaradzki, J. (2022). '"We Are Also Here" – Spiritual Care Practitioners' Experiences of the COVID-19 Pandemic: A Qualitative Study from Poland', *Journal of Religion and Health* 61. DOI: 10.1007/s10943-021-01492-3.

JW (Jehovah's Witnesses). (2019). *2019 Coordinators' Committee Report – Supporting Our Brothers When Disasters Strike*. Accessible online at URL: https://www.jw.org/en/news/jw/region/global/support-when-epidemics-disasters-strike/.

JW. (2020). *2020 Governing Body Update #4*. Accessible online at URL: https://
    www.jw.org/finder?wtlocale=E&docid=702020283&srcid=share.
JW. (n.d.). 'Are Jehovah's Witnesses Opposed to Vaccination?'. Accessible
    online at URL: https://www.jw.org/en/jehovahs-witnesses/faq/jw-vaccines-
    immunization/.
Torres-Pruñonosa, J., M. A. Plaza-Navas, and S. Brown. (2022). 'Jehovah's
    Witnesses Adoption of Digitally-Mediated Services during COVID-19
    Pandemic'. *Cogent Social Services* 8 (1). DOI:10.1080/23311886.2022.2071034.

27

How one Jehovah's Witness community negotiated the ride of the 'pale horse'

Gary Perkins

The railway town of Carnforth in England developed in the nineteenth century, but its location, nestled beside an area of outstanding natural beauty between Morecambe Bay and the Lake District, is far from ordinary. This being the case, when reports from China of an outbreak of coronavirus hit the news in early 2020 this probably did not pique the interest of most Carnforth residents. After all, as one resident stated, 'These sorts of things don't happen here, do they?'

One local religious group that does take an unusual interest in international news reports, however, are Jehovah's Witnesses. Believing we live deep in the last days Christ foretold, many in the Carnforth congregation 'keep on the watch' as wars, famines, earthquakes and pestilences in the world fulfil expectations relating to the 'sign of the times', a precursor to Armageddon and better times ahead when God's Kingdom establishes a paradise on earth (Mt. 24; 16.3; Lk. 21.11; Rev. 16.14, 16; 21.3, 4). Some wondered, might disease, the fourth and pale horse of Revelation chapter 6, now be about to threaten the peace of this semi-rural community?

On 11 March 2020, a Witness engaging in his ministry in a nearby village chatted with an NHS worker. The man, polite though not especially interested in discussing the Bible, expressed genuine anxiety at the Witness visiting elderly and vulnerable people at this time. The visitor thanked him for his concern but explained that, since the UK government had not yet hinted that coronavirus had reached here, he was happy to continue. However, just two days after the conversation, on 13 March, the International Governing Body of Jehovah's Witnesses informed congregation elders in Britain that, with immediate effect, all public witnessing including door-to-door visits, home Bible studies and use of literature carts at strategic public locations was to end. Also, shortly thereafter, Kingdom Hall meetings were to be replaced by online meetings in an 'unprecedented' move taken due to both respect for human life and international public health concerns.

Although it would not be until 23 March 2020 that the UK government announced the need for an immediate national lockdown, neither the NHS worker nor Jehovah's Witnesses were being alarmist in showing concern at the arrival of the pandemic which sadly would cause so much human tragedy. Indeed, the congregation soon became painfully aware of the danger when Mandy, a local Witness and NHS nurse, tested positive for six weeks before slowly recovering.

Witnesses faced the same issues that challenged all faiths: What could be done practically to help individuals in the local congregation survive the pandemic? How could the mental health of fellow believers, particularly the elderly and those living alone in isolated locations facing prolonged lockdown periods, be maintained? Could the congregation somehow stay united throughout in loving thoughts, words and deeds? And what about its concern for the wider local community, including the commission to preach the good news of God's Kingdom, as Witnesses understand it? (Mt. 24.14)

Preparing and adapting to lockdown measures

In preparation for lockdown, on 19 March 2020 Jehovah's Witnesses became the first religious group in the area to adopt online meetings. Most of the Witnesses had long used the JW Library App on their tablets at meetings and in their ministry. Additionally, an online meeting platform was recommended for their religious services. Consequently, once this had been installed on their computers, tablets or smartphones, few had difficulty adapting. With minimal assistance, older ones, including some who previously resisted technology, quickly mastered accessing meetings, putting their virtual hands up and turning on their cameras and microphones to comment. Video-conferencing proved a blessing in keeping the congregation together over the next two years while illustrating the true flavour of an international brotherhood as public talks were occasionally given online by speakers from Africa, America, Brazil, India and Japan. With interested individuals often visiting alongside Witnesses whose health complaints might prevent them from attending some Kingdom Hall meetings, attendances were consistently high. However, all recognized these somehow lacked the intimacy and feel of Kingdom Hall meetings.

Attitude to authority

Jehovah's Witnesses sincerely believe that it is their responsibility before God to follow government regulations. They follow what the Bible recommends, namely to 'be obedient to governments and authorities' (Tit. 3.1). They also respect the authority of governments under which they live, in harmony with the Bible's command: 'Let every person be in subjection to the superior authorities' (Rom. 13.1, NWT). Accordingly, all complied with lockdown requirements, which they considered evidence of a benevolent government. Since calls to frequently wash hands, wear face masks and perform social distancing in public had already been promoted by the Witnesses' Governing Body, these were readily supported. But when the government's lockdown and guidelines eventually eased, Witnesses remained cautious.

Witnesses are not opposed to vaccination and view this as a personal decision for each Christian to make (Gal. 6.5). After the arrival of Covid vaccinations in Britain in December 2020, most Witnesses readily accepted these and expressed appreciation for the generous help of the UK government and NHS. This was especially the case after the Governing Body indicated that the majority of Witness deaths from Covid worldwide had occurred before vaccines became available; in sharp contrast, 99 per cent of the world headquarters staff had chosen to be vaccinated with complications proving to be minimal. A handful of local Witnesses remained unvaccinated, but their decision continued to be respected, with none showing signs of promoting anti-vax conspiracy theories.

Coping mechanisms

Witness congregations have always been subdivided into groups overseen by elders, a set-up which lent itself well to surviving the pandemic. Duties of the elders include caring for the pastoral needs of each person in their respective groups, as the Bible says: 'You ought to know positively the appearance of your flock' (Prov. 27.23). In Carnforth, there are six groups of approximately 15–18 people. Each is led by an overseer, a fellow elder and a ministerial servant, who offer spiritual nourishment. Initially, online meetings were held on a group level until all became familiar with videoconferencing and meetings were restored congregationally.

During the pandemic, practical help included providing transportation for those living in isolated areas, delivering food supplies or ensuring online deliveries were set up. Enquiries were made for those facing economic hardship because of being laid off from work during the early weeks of lockdown with the financially comfortable using their resources to fund those struggling. Congregation elders took the lead in supporting elderly and sick Jehovah's Witnesses by ringing them by phone or by simply speaking with them online, and they and their wives wrote cards and sent flowers. Additionally, to the extent that local laws eventually allowed, short visits were made wearing masks and respecting Covid protocols.

Individuals who might have struggled were supported even more when early government lockdown rules eased to allow isolated individuals to become included in family 'bubbles'. An example is Dawn, who was supported by Rosalind with meals, transport, shopping, doctors' appointments and in claiming benefits she was entitled to receive after her husband John had tragically died early during lockdown. Likewise, Jo, a single mother with two sons with special needs, became part of the Walker family bubble, an arrangement that proved mutually advantageous. Becky, a young single Witness, provided heroic support for Shirley, an aged Witness widow with terminal cancer. And Sam and Edna, an elderly couple in declining health, received regular calls, visits and travel help from Brian, Pat and others. How much comfort was brought to members of the congregation because of loving measures initiated and promoted by local elders on their behalf! (2 Cor. 1.5-7)

In addition to organizationally arranged Sunday morning and Thursday evening meetings, the Congregation spontaneously developed daily and monthly activities to respond to the general challenge of social isolation that brothers and sisters experienced. These included online daily 10 a.m. meetups to share discussion of a scriptural text, connect, encourage, engage and strengthen individuals. Also, online congregational social events were arranged, including a fun monthly general knowledge quiz and regular online tours, which connected attendees worldwide and attracted non-Witness friends also, including subjects as diverse as the British Museum, Oxford University, the life of Isaac Newton and the history of Jehovah's Witnesses in Nazi Germany.

Thinking outside the box

The pivotal date on the 2020 Witness calendar was 7 April, which marked the yearly Memorial of Christ's death. Normally Witnesses visit every home in their area to extend invitations. This year, instead, Witnesses phoned, texted and emailed friends, business contacts and those who had previously responded favourably to their house-to-house ministry to invite these to an online Memorial with attendees exhorted in advance to purchase appropriate wine and make their own unleavened bread. These efforts were reciprocated with an online Memorial attendance of 127, just four below their record ever Kingdom Hall attendance.

As the pandemic dragged on, individuals considered what else could be done to reach the wider community. Denied their public face, Witnesses adapted their approach to evangelism. The daily text meetups morphed into a daily ministry arrangement aimed at reaching all suffering from loneliness, dejection and anxiety, as Witnesses wrote letters and cards, spending considerable sums of their own money on stamps to reach people in houses they would previously have visited in person, addressing these to 'The Resident', since data protection laws prevent collating a database of named householders.

Letters showed concern for people's welfare, offered hope and encouraged prayer, inviting receivers to make contact by letter or phone and visit online meetings. Themes included discussion of the purpose of life, why God allows suffering, the hope of a resurrection for those who had lost loved ones in death and the 'good news of the Kingdom'. Others were related to current news items including ecological damage, climate change, corruption in government, selfishness and war, and the pandemic itself, all richly illustrative, from the Witness perspective, of Christ's 'sign of the times' and the better world to follow. Most seemed gifted at letter writing, able to convey complex religious ideas briefly and effectively, but one older Witness admitted being hesitant, never having written a letter in her life. With a little help, she wrote a letter and never looked back.

Residents often cut short Witnesses in their door-to-door visits, whereas letters enable a biblical theme to be progressed to a meaningful conclusion. Admiration, curiosity or even annoyance probably ensured that most letters were read in full, with a more thorough message likely being delivered to the public than has been accomplished before. Public responses varied, with several residents writing to compliment this example of Christian outreach with one person commenting that Witnesses 'express themselves better in writing than at the doorstep'. And a few replied respectfully asking no further letters be sent.

Some Witnesses initiated conversations by phone, enjoying the instant response unavailable in letter writing while engaging in constructive conversations and being surprised by how relaxed residents were. Others added stickers to their front doors or car windows – something they do not ordinarily do – making people aware of JW.org and, unprompted, Witness children painted positive Bible verses on pebbles left in public places. Finally, those whose interest had waned were recontacted, sometimes with positive results. Andy and Anne-Marie, for instance, admitted that the pandemic was a 'wake-up call'. They welcomed an online Bible Study and joined our virtual meetings including the regular daily ministry meet-ups. On 24 July 2021, after government regulations allowed limited social contact, both were baptized using an outside bathing pool specially hired for the occasion.

In these various ways, what had started as a daily personal preoccupation for individual congregation believers to survive, slowly developed to become a group challenge, a congregational accomplishment and then a compassionate desire to reach out to all in our local community.

Review and lessons learned

So how did the congregation fare during the first two years of Covid, leading up until June 2022 when cart witnessing returned in Carnforth, with all forms of public ministry being reinstated other than door-to-door witnessing? By this time twenty-two members of the congregation had contracted Covid at some point. Thankfully, its effects, while unpleasant, had likely been curtailed due to vaccination and none have died from the virus.

After displaying an abundance of caution during the pandemic's first two years, it came as a shock when the Governing Body announced the return of Kingdom Hall meetings from April 2022. Although other religious groups had returned to in-person church services some considerable time before, by the Spring of 2022 local infections were known to be spiralling. However, probably due to vaccinations, by this time the variant forms of the virus posed significantly less of a threat to public health than they once had.

Meetings continued in a hybrid form, with the option to attend in person at the ultra-sanitized Kingdom Hall wearing a mask or watch online. Those displaying cold or flu-like symptoms, or who had been exposed to, or tested positive for Covid within the past ten days were asked to watch online. That apart, it was stressed that it was a matter of personal choice whether one attended in person or online and that such decisions should be respected, which they were, with 102 attending our first hybrid meeting on 3 April 2022, consisting of 51 in person and 51 online. Attendances since have increasingly tilted in favour of Kingdom Hall meetings, with one plus from Covid, it seems, being that those with genuine health complaints that once prevented involvement in meetings are now catered for. Previously there was only a phone tie-in, whereas now they can hear, see, comment and associate.

Throughout, Witnesses expressed indebtedness to their Governing Body for providing swift and unambiguous direction without undue control. Most importantly, Witnesses believe that their ultra-sensitive approach minimized loss of life among the public and their brotherhood alike. This concern was mirrored by tireless local 'shepherds' whose caring attitude energized Witnesses when spirits might otherwise have flagged. Consequently, local believers retained focus in their lives, kept united in their worship and remained true to their name and purpose as Witnesses to their God, Jehovah. This in turn heightened their desire to compassionately show concern for the spiritual and physical needs of all suffering in the local community, especially those seemingly without hope. During the crisis, Witnesses could be seen caring practically for their non-Witness neighbours too, with some giving generously to local food banks.

Probably the most valuable lesson learned since most people in Carnforth knew someone who had died from Covid is that – wherever we live – no one can be safe when disease, the pale horse of Revelation chapter 6, rides. A stark reminder to cherish our precious and fragile life, using it now to love God with our whole heart, soul and mind, and to love our neighbours as ourselves (Mk. 12.29-31).

Reference

New World Bible Translation Committee. (2013). *New World Translation of the Holy Scriptures*. Walkill, NY: Watchtower Bible and Tract Society of New York.

28

Practising my Christian Science faith during the Covid-19 pandemic

Shirley Paulson

When the highly contagious Covid-19 was approaching my town, I probably asked the same questions most people did. What do I really believe about God in the context of such a disease? What's the most loving and unselfish thing to do concerning my family, neighbours and the world? What's the best way to protect myself? Identifying myself as a practising adherent of Christian Science implies a pro-active, religious response to whatever impacts my health and well-being as well as the health and well-being of others. My custom is to turn to a prayerful and mentally disciplined approach to hurtful physical and emotional phenomena. Some of my prayers have resulted in extraordinarily wonderful healing experiences, but other prayers have concluded in disappointment.

I think everybody would prefer God's immediate removal of the effects of disease without the need for medical intervention if that was possible. Christian Scientists usually hold that expectation, but people often presume Christian Scientists believe in magic, or that their church membership entitles them to divine favours. A Christian Scientist would probably explain that healing requires humble biblically guided prayer, reasoning, disciplined thought and a conviction that God's care – based on a law of divine Love – continues under every circumstance.

The Christian Science community

I should mention that the Christian Science Church plays a role in these decisions, but not as much as conscience and experience do. The church offers spiritual guidance and encouragement, but fortunately there is no biblical or church mandate to forgo medical intervention. In all candour, there is also some unspoken pressure from fellow Christian Scientists to seek healing through spiritual means rather than medical means because a healing through spiritual means alone implies a heightened level of spirituality. But I believe an increasing number of practising Christian Scientists view these decisions more humbly as personal responsibilities, rather than proof of one's spiritual qualifications.

Having spent my childhood and adult years with this prayer-first approach to illness, accidents and life problems, I brought this life experience to the onset of the pandemic. Here are the first topics I addressed in my prayers:

1 Confronting panic by prayerfully staying calm myself and for others
2 Discerning contagious mental elements associated with the pandemic, such as fear, global anger in politics, economic disparity and police violence
3 Awareness of the increasing importance of interpersonal, community and global relationships
4 Seeking spiritual guidance for response to the unknown behaviour of this disease
5 Asking what I could do for others who are either afraid or suffering

The foundation of my prayer and conviction is the timeless message of the Bible and Mary Baker Eddy's interpretation of it. She identifies the continuity of God's presence and action in terms of an eternal science. I think of it the same way we might imagine the action of the ocean. Storms can produce high winds, lightning and dangerous seas, but far below the surface, the calm remains steady. This pandemic was a new and ferocious storm, blowing in new questions and new prayers for me. But my *practices* remained the same, based on underlying laws of divine order, such as these biblical messages:

Bless the LORD, O my soul, and do not forget all his benefits – who forgives all your iniquity, who heals all your diseases, who redeems your life from the Pit, who crowns you with steadfast love and mercy.

(Ps.103.2-4, NRSV)

But strive first for the kingdom of God and his righteousness, and all these things will be given to you as well.

(Mt. 6.33, NRSV)

Then Jesus called the twelve together and gave them power and authority over all demons and to cure diseases, and he sent them out to proclaim the kingdom of God and to heal.

(Lk. 9.1-2, NRSV)

The difference with a pandemic

Even with these promises, the arrival of the pandemic pushed me deeper. Where *is* God in the midst of a disease that threatens the whole world? Violence, disease and the injustice of random chaos of the world contradicts God's presence, goodness and empowerment. The daily news of Covid dangers and frustrations in our collective efforts to handle it forced me to decide frequently what I was leaning on and why. And deep down I think it comes down to: either God is all good and all-powerful, or God is not.

I think of prayer as the willingness to align myself with the underlying reality of God's goodness, despite my own reluctance. I allow Christ to turn me, as in repentance, from my own limited view. Although this change of perspective removes the blame for evil from God, the obvious danger in this is the ease with which I could kid myself about the severity of the peril for others and even myself with a blind eye towards the serious threats of disease.

But honest prayer helps me discern a little better *how* God is caring for humanity. Instead of blindly denying the situation, an agreement with God's capacity to empower us and to love us orients me towards what can be done. For instance, I heard on some news reports how there was a marked correlation in the intensity of the disease for those with heightened anxiety compared with those who remained calmer. Quiet faith – a kind of spiritual immunity – helps one hear God's guidance better. It also became clear early on that political and social/cultural views seemed to drive reactions as much as or more than medical advice. This growing awareness of the impact of human choices impressed upon me the significance of Jesus's teaching that compliance with the two 'great commandments' (loving God and loving one's neighbour) will enable all of us to live – literally. (See Lk. 10.25-29.) I could see better than ever before why loving one's neighbour was so relevant to life itself. In a global pandemic, everyone counts.

In a sense, the fact that this was a disease that could impact anyone in the world shifted the powerbase even more significantly for me. Although rich and powerful people had more options to choose from than the poor and politically weak, no human rulers had the power to halt the disease in their own countries, and in some cases, even in their own bodies. Regardless of state rulings, individuals always had choices for how to think and pray. The nature of a global pandemic heightened my awareness that global interdependence had become the centre of my faith-struggles. How should I think about others who make choices contrary to my own? I cannot change them, and they have no power to make me think one way or another. But knowing I have access to Divine guidance in my unique situation at any time, I know others do too. Like the availability of a principle of mathematics, everyone has access to a unique solution, even when our problems are different from one another.

Individual responsibility or community priorities?

One of the characteristics I inherited from the origins of my Christian Science faith tradition is an emphasis on my individual responsibility and salvation. Mary Baker Eddy, the nineteenth-century founder of Christian Science, was raised in a pious Puritan (Christian) tradition where individualism reigned over social dependence, and this moral and spiritual integrity permeates her teaching. While her followers are taught not to blame other people or things for their troubles – society at large, health or simply happenstance – we tend to search within for whatever would interfere with our salvation (immediate and future physical or moral healing).

Personal responsibility is a good thing. But when access to Covid-19 vaccinations finally arrived, the fact that my choices were not solely about me magnified. My thoughts about others mattered in significant ways. A verse from Paul's letter to the Romans encourages the consideration of others' needs and the well-being of others: 'I say to everyone among you not to think of yourself more highly than you ought to think, ... For as in one body we have many members, and not all the members have the same function, so we, who are many, are one body in Christ, and individually we are members one of another' (Rom. 12. 3-5, NRSV). Would I opt out of the vaccines because I 'think of myself more highly' than others who don't practise religion as I do? Or, am I part of the larger global body?

Furthermore, a Bible verse pushed in another line of questioning. 'For God did not give us a spirit of cowardice, but rather a spirit of power and of love and of self-discipline' (2 Tim. 1.7, NRSV). Even with vaccines, the urgency to remain faithful and to give my best persisted, but would the vaccine make it easier to hide behind social pressure and ease up on my prayers? Another complication for some Christian Scientists was the fact that so many of them have never been vaccinated or taken medication, so the fear of the vaccine was greater than fear of the disease. Would they find excuses to avoid the vaccine because they were truly afraid of it?

These are no small questions. To stay faithful to my highest beliefs comes with a struggle, so I understand why so many of my fellow Christian Scientists from around the world reacted within a wide range of responses regarding mask-wearing, social distancing and vaccines. Many were praying earnestly; some were fearful, some rather dismissive about the whole situation and others searching for their own direction.

I thought of Mary Baker Eddy's brief letter to her adult son who had not wanted to pay for the required vaccination of his own son at school. She wrote to him in 1900, 'I am sorry that you have entered suit on the question of vacinating [sic] your child or children … If it was my child I should let them vacinate [sic] him and then with Christian Science I would prevent its harming the health of my child' (Eddy, 1900). This letter is reasoned and modest, and it is consistent with the teaching in Eddy's Church *Manual*, where she wrote, 'Christian Science can only be practised according to the Golden Rule: "All things whatsoever ye would that men should do to you, do ye even so to them"' (Mt. 7.12, quoted from Eddy, 1895, 42). These two points grounded my own decision to prioritize attentiveness and care for others and to find my own protection from both vaccines and disease through my faith in God, even while I wore masks and got the vaccine.

The congregational element

Christian Science practice takes place both privately and within a congregational context. The deepest prayers probably take place within the quiet of one's own sacred space and time. But church-sponsored activities, such as services, lectures, Reading Rooms, religious periodicals and teaching, are also designed to support and strengthen the individual's spiritual growth. During the pandemic, when governments requested church closures, some Christian Science churches did adapt to online services, and others encouraged their congregants to connect temporarily with other Christian Science communities. A few stretched the local suggestions as far as they could by holding in-person services and not requiring masks for attendance. Christian Scientists observe Eucharist and baptism in a spiritual sense without physical implements. That is, they seek communion with God in their hearts, and they acknowledge the baptismal cleansing of sin through the Holy Spirit. Therefore, the lack of ritual acts in physical buildings were no impediment to these sacraments. But without being together, I did wonder how effectively we were engaging in them.

Surprisingly, one of the most important questions that the pandemic brought to my attention was how to evaluate both the beneficial and harmful effects of religious practices, particularly those I was most familiar with. These three concerned me. First, surely prayers that heal disease are beneficial. But at what point do people determine they are not up to the spiritual maturity required in the context of a pandemic? Seeking a divine source of calm trust brings peace to tense situations, but when does the calm trust cover up a bland denial of both the individual and global needs at hand? Second, taking responsibility to pray for the health and safety of everyone surely adds some level of support to all those praying alongside their communities. When the nature of the disease is deadly, the prayer must necessarily confront fear. But when the disease is also highly contagious, we cannot afford to address only our personal and family situations at the neglect of the fears and concerns of everyone around us. Third, the medical uncertainties and contradictions, as well as the political pressures, that surfaced during the tense months of the pandemic escalation highlighted the need for alternative assurances, such as an abiding sense of divine presence. But blind faith in spiritual treatment is no more efficacious than a placebo. The real need for spiritual clarity, strength and authority sharpened for me.

What changed, or what have I learned?

As life experiences change, so does the nature of my faith. My habit of gratitude is a reminder to acknowledge God's power to adjust things for good. It is like the depth of the ocean that remains calm during the storm. But my faith in some people, institutions and ways of doing things has been shaken. As usual, such stirring results in more lessons in maturity. I notice spiritual and moral improvements in myself and others, but I also notice weaknesses undetected before. I am sobered to realize the breadth and depth of the world's convulsions. But Eddy asserts that 'the awful daring of sin destroys sin, and foreshadows the triumph of truth. God will overturn, until "He come whose right it is"' (Eddy [1875] 1934, 223).

I am humbled to acknowledge that there is a divine law of Love that will always be impelling and compelling the world to thrive, operating even in the darkest hours of the pandemic exacerbated by racial violence, economic instability and political polemics. I am inspired by the examples of others who found resilience, grace, healing and love. I am convinced God never sent the darkness, but that God loves all of us enough to show us the way forward. I hope I have gained enough humility to take hold of these lessons and keep learning, even after the pressure has abated.

References

Eddy, M. B. (1895). *Church Manual of the First Church of Christ, Scientist, in Boston, Massachusetts*. Boston: The First Church of Christ, Scientist.

Eddy, M. B. (1900). Letter from Mary Baker Eddy to her son, L02130. Boston MA: Mary Baker Eddy Library.

Eddy, M. B. ([1875] 1934). *Science and Health with Key to the Scriptures*. Boston: The First Church of Christ, Scientist.

29

Personal experiences of the Christian Science faith during Covid

Susan Searle

Australia has faced many challenges in the past few years. Wildfires decimated our eastern coastal region including the area where my family and I live. When Covid hit it all seemed too much to take in. We were still trying to mentally and physically process and recover from the devastation of the wildfires. Like many people of faith the wildfires, Covid and now floods left me asking why this had happened and how does my concept of an all-loving, all-good God, as Christian Science teaches, fit into all this?

Previous healing experiences and healthcare choices

I am a lifelong Christian Scientist and have relied on the practicality of its teaching to address many of the problems that come up in everyday life, such as finding a home, employment, relationship problems and healthcare. The Golden Rule (Lk. 6.31) and the two great commandments, 'to love the Lord your God with all your heart and with all your soul and with all your mind' and 'Love your neighbour as yourself' (Mt. 22.36-39), have guided my prayers for myself and my community previously and they form the basis of my prayers in regard to the Covid pandemic. Sometimes I wonder what good my prayers for others and our world are when the situation seems so overwhelming.

However, I feel empowered and hopeful when I remember that the power is not within me but rather the outcome of the power and presence of God's grace. My prayers are an acknowledgement of this.

My healthcare choice, in most cases, has been to rely on prayerful treatment as explained in Christian Science. I have found it an effective form of treatment for less serious as well as serious issues. This treatment acknowledges God as omnipotent, omnipresent, omniscient, good and our inseparability from this goodness as his creation made in his image and likeness (Gen. 1.27-31). There are seven synonyms used in Christian Science which help me to understanding the quality and vastness of God and how he is expressed in our lives. They are Life, Truth, Love, Mind, Soul, Spirit and Principle (Eddy, [1875] 1934: 465). God is also acknowledged as the Father and Mother of all. If I have felt the need to use medical means I have been grateful for the care, dedication and compassion of the medical staff. The global experience with the Covid pandemic has highlighted their dedication and compassion to the world at large.

In my experience Christian Science treatment results not only in an improved physical condition but a greater sense of harmony and well-being as a result of understanding and feeling the power and influence of divine Love. Often a healing has resulted in an uncovering of a misapprehension of the nature of God and my identity, accompanied by a change in character. For example a long-standing skin cancer diminished in size and totally disappeared when I understood more clearly that beauty is a spiritual quality of Soul (God) and not dependent on body. It made me ask myself the question, What am I seeing? I realized I needed to be less critical of myself and others and claim for each of us our individual identity as God's beautiful spiritual idea.

Some healings happen quickly, others have taken much longer. The choice has always been mine and fortunately I have been supported by family and my church community, whatever path I have chosen for my healthcare.

Why I chose to be vaccinated

In Australia vaccination was not compulsory. However, the substantial restriction placed on those unvaccinated made life difficult. Previously my choice in regard to vaccination has been to rely solely on my understanding of God's law of harmony for my protection. I prayed and listened to God's guidance for some time before I made my decision to be vaccinated for Covid. A number of factors influenced me. I felt the fear of my family and the wider community to the transmission of Covid was much more intense. I also volunteered with a homeless organization and these people were considered more vulnerable to Covid. I chose not to exacerbate the fears of others as a way of practising loving my neighbour, and the Golden Rule, as Jesus urges us to do. The founder of Christian Science, Mary Baker Eddy, recommended that 'Where vaccination is compulsory, let your children be vaccinated, and see that your mind is in such a state that by your prayers vaccination will do the children no harm' (Eddy ([1913] 1941: 344). Although I chose to be vaccinated for Covid I continue praying for protection from contagion for myself and others.

Before Covid I had completed training as a hospital pastoral care volunteer but was not able to continue with the work due to a requirement to be vaccinated according to the National Standards immunization programme. I understand life as sustained and controlled by God and I give all power to God. Although I acknowledge the benefits of both the National Standard immunization programme and now the Covid vaccination programme to alleviate the suffering of others and offer them protection from disease, I do not accept that vaccinations have the power to benefit me. Nor do I fear they can harm me, whether that harm is associated with a substance, conspiracy or government control. I have found placing my faith in the practical understanding of God's law of love for all of his creation more effective in maintaining harmony in my life, including the protection from disease. However, I now see vaccination as something required to enable me to go on and bless others in a volunteer capacity. It does not distract from my commitment to practise my faith or make my prayers less effective.

I had an opportunity to put into practice what I had been declaring in my prayers about freedom from side effects. After my first vaccination I experienced severe side effects including chest pain, high temperature and blurred vision. I had a choice to make. Was I going to call an ambulance or rely on Christian Science prayerful treatment? I chose the latter. However, I did ring my daughter-in-law and ask her to come and be with me. When my daughter-in-law arrived, approximately ten minutes later, I was on the phone with a Christian Science practitioner. She shared passages from the Bible and *Science and Health with Key to the Scriptures*, the textbook of Christian Science, which assisted me to overcome fear and focus consciousness more on the authority of the law of God's love than in material conditions. As a result, all side effects subsided, and I was very grateful for this evidence of God's universal law of care and protection. This was an interesting and growing experience for me. It tested my faith. I had previously seen evidence of God's law of unfailing love at work in my life and others and this experience confirmed I could trust in the reliability of this law no matter what the circumstance.

God causes only good

A God that is all good does not bring suffering upon his creation, so I don't see illness, or any inharmony in our lives, as inflicted by God. In Jer. 29.1 (NIV) we read 'I know the plans I have for you, declares the Lord, plans to prosper you and not to harm you, plans to give you hope and a future'. Jesus often made a connection between healing and consciousness through his forgiveness of sins or commendation of people's faith but he did not judge or condemn them. Rather Jesus's sense of compassion corrected their sense of separation from Love, from good, and the effect was healing (Mt. 9.2, 20-22; Mk 10.46-52; Lk. 7.36-50; Jn 8.3-11). As God is all good there is no power opposing God's goodness, no place or time when God's goodness, love and life is absent. Therefore, Covid is not a punishment from God but an opportunity to grow spiritually. Just as my healing of skin cancer was an opportunity to gain a better spiritual sense of beauty and feel the healing effect of the presence of God's love, Covid has impelled individuals, churches and society to think differently; be more creative; and to re-evaluate what is important. An understanding of God as all good has encouraged me to look for good, or the evidence of the influence of God, in others and in difficult life situations such as Covid.

Churches, businesses, governments and individuals have had to be more creative in how they function. I see this openness to new possibilities and the creative thinking required as the expression of God as Mind. In my own family I saw evidence of this opening up opportunities that previously were not considered possible. The requirement to isolate and work from home caused the re-evaluation of priorities in the career-home balance. It enabled a mother to spend more time at home with her infant when previously the child would have spent long hours in childcare and the mother many hours in travel. Mother and child have developed a closer relationship, and both are happier. It also made it possible for my son, who was experiencing housing difficulties, to stay with me as distance would not restrict his ability to work.

For some the requirement to isolate caused hardship as a result of loneliness and separation from family. For others, it gave them the opportunity to re-evaluate the importance of spending time with family and being active through walking and appreciating nature. Initially it provided me with valuable time and quiet space for self-reflection and to come to terms with what was happening in the world. Another friend said it helped her appreciate that she really did like spending time with others and encouraged her to do this more often in the future. Later, the blessing of more time with my son helped us both gain insight into the problems, interests and joys of each other's lives and share the mutual enjoyment of walking in nature. My grandchildren, like most of the children in Australia during lockdown, needed to be home-schooled, and this helped our communities better appreciate the teaching profession. This was also true for shop assistants, and others in caring professions such as nursing, childcare and aged care. I am hopeful that this new-found appreciation will transfer into government policy.

There is some debate over the effect of Covid on the environment. Lockdowns and work from home arrangements saw a decrease in the use of cars and other transport, resulting in less air pollution but this benefit was only short-lived. However, a study by Dr Quentin Maire, Dr Eric Fu and Associate Professor Jenny Chesters (2020 sec. 2, par. 3; sec. 3, par. 2) showed that since the pandemic climate change is now the major concern of Australians and there is an increased community expectation for governments to act on the problem. This has been reflected in our recent federal elections that returned a change in government and an increase in seats for the Greens and independents running on addressing climate change.

I see God as the agent for change for good in the world through spiritual inspiration working in individuals and the community to bring a change in thought for good. I understand this as the Christ, 'God speaking to the human consciousness' and this is what animated Jesus (Eddy, [1875] 1934: 332). Mary Baker Eddy states, 'God is the lawmaker, but He is not the author of barbarous codes' (Eddy, [1875] 1934: 381).

Adapting Church to Covid restrictions

Our church, like many other organizations, needed to adapt. My prayers to find solutions embraced all religious organizations as we all tried to find practical steps to meet the needs of our congregations; address isolation; and comfort those who may be experiencing illness, bereavement or financial hardship due to the pandemic. I acknowledged that God meets the needs of all humanity, including those of other faiths or no faith, as a loving, spiritual, Father and Mother of all. Before Covid my branch church already held hybrid services with the congregation attending either in-person or by conference telephone call. We found this met the needs of our congregation by allowing those with no transportation or living long distances from the church to still feel part of our church family. The Covid lockdowns compelled us to expand this service to include video conferencing; screen sharing of the lesson sermon, hymns and prayers; and to improve the quality of the music. The true function of church is not contained within a building or place but is the coming together of individuals who lovingly support each other's developing understanding of Truth and the presence and operation of Love.

This desire and practice of love has a solid foundation and the storms of human existence, such as Covid, cannot undermine it.

The resources created by the Mother Church, the Christian Science denomination's organizational head, together with other resources, helped us to improve the quality of our online services. This continues to bless those who join our hybrid services by phone or video conference today.

What I learnt

Covid provided a catalyst in my spiritual growth. I witnessed the practical demonstration of what church looks like when we embrace a more spiritual concept of it. Although I love my church building and community, I understand more profoundly now that we can still maintain that sense of a mutually supportive congregation even when we need to move away from the old ways of doing things. The healing I experience from the side effects of the Covid vaccine gave me confidence to continue to rely on the teachings of Christian Science. Covid prompted me to research deeply Mary Baker Eddy's writing in regard to vaccinations and this together with my prayers, and self-reflection has resulted in a more open approach to vaccinations in general.

During the Covid epidemic, and particularly during lockdowns, I saw more people showing concern for the vulnerable and finding new and creative ways to come together and love their community. This I understand as evidence of God's love in action.

References

Chester, J., E. Jun Fu, Q. Maire, 'Australians More Concerned about Climate Change than Covid-19'. Accessible online at URL: https://pursuit.unimelb.edu.au/articles/australians-more-concerned-about-climate-change-than-covid-19.

Eddy, M. B. ([1875] 1934). *Science and Health with Key to the Scriptures*. Boston: The First Church of Christ, Scientist.

Eddy, M. B. ([1913] 1941). *First Church of Christ, Scientist, and Miscellany*. Boston: The First Church of Christ, Scientist.

30

Covid and Theology

Dan Cohn-Sherbok

Twenty years ago I edited a collection of responses to the theological dilemmas posed by the Holocaust: *Holocaust Theology: A Reader* (University of Exeter Press, 2002). Since the end of the Second World War both Jewish and Christian thinkers have wrested with the central problem of the Holocaust: Where was God when six million died? If God is all-good and all-powerful, how could he have permitted this terrible tragedy to take place? The aim of the book was to provide a panoramic survey of the responses of over one hundred Jewish and Christian theologians.

The Covid Pandemic and the World's Religions poses similar theological difficulties. Where was God during Covid? How could he have allowed so many to suffer and die? As we have seen, contributors to this volume have provided a wide range of responses to this haunting question. In the Introduction, Christopher Lewis points out that in previous centuries it was common for religious thinkers to view plagues as caused by God. In their view, God was sending believers to paradise, whereas non-believers were being punished for their lack of belief.

In this volume, however, no one has expressed such a view. None of the contributors contend that Covid is in any sense a punishment, no matter how they understand divine reality. Instead they emphatically reject such a suggestion. David Zucker in the Judaism chapter, for example, stresses that there are laws of nature – such as tsunamis and earthquakes – that result in human suffering. It is not the divine will that brings such disasters about. Hence, Covid should not in any sense be perceived as a divinely ordained punishment for human misbehaviour.

For some contributors there is simply no way of providing a comprehensive theodicy. Oliver Leaman, in the Judaism chapter, for example, argues that

Judaism does not have a clear and definitive answer to the problem of evil. In this context he cites the book of Job, which does not seek to explain why humans suffer. According to the book's author, God's ways are beyond human comprehension.

Other contributors, however, seek in different ways to provide various explanations of divine presence in the face of Covid. Claire Amos, for example, writing about Christianity, stresses that according to the Christian faith God is deeply involved both in the suffering of Christ and of the world. In this way God, through the passion of Jesus, shares deeply in human pain. Camille Kaminski Lewis stresses that it is vital to remember the ways in which Covid has challenged us. If we remember the struggles and how we coped with this crisis, we can underline God's care, our persistence and the best practices in the face of a pandemic. In remembering, we can have hope.

For many Muslims Covid is viewed in relation to divine providence. In the Islam chapter Usama Hasan cites Caliph Omar who viewed everything as the decree of God. In this regard he refers to a common Muslim saying that the world is a place of test. Whether good or bad things happen to us, they are a test from God: in good times, to see if we will be grateful; in bad times, to see if we will be patient. Yet as Farhana Mayer points out in the same chapter, it should not be overlooked that Covid emerged due to human activity. The pandemic, she writes, is arguably the result of bad husbandry, poor hygiene standards in wet markets or mistakes in dubious laboratory manipulations.

Turning to Hinduism, such theological speculation does not appear to be a primary concern. Anantanand Rambachan notes that significant attention does not appear to have been paid to the theological perplexities poised by Covid in Hindu communities. Covid has not dismissed faith among Hindus, he writes, because God is not held to be responsible. According to Rambachan, the Hindu response to Covid has been largely pragmatic and empirical. Echoing this view, Shaunaka Rishi Das and Utsa Bose in the same chapter write that there was hardly a voice that blamed God. Rather it was understood that the pandemic was due to our failure. By contrast, the Supreme was the shelter, the source of strength to endure and the source of joy amidst distress.

Unlike these faiths that wrestle in various ways with the problem of suffering and divine providence, Buddhism has a different focus. Peter Harvey, in his contribution to the Buddhism chapter, stresses that various forms of illness are an inevitable aspect of life. Covid has reminded us of this reality. For Buddhists, calmly reflecting on this aspect of human life can have a beneficial meditative effect. Continuing this discussion, Bogodá Seelawimala emphasizes that the Buddha serves as a means of confronting such suffering. The Buddha, he writes, was a great compassionate doctor and pointed out that disease is an inevitable part of our lives. Facing Covid, Buddhists should take refuge in his teachings.

Shinto theology adopts a very different approach to the problem of Covid. Taishi Kato explains that the Covid pandemic should be viewed in relation to the spiritual realm of the *kami*. Both good and evil workings exist for human beings, he writes. Considering *kami*'s work in the current pandemic situation, it is believed that the pestilence epidemic is also *kami*'s work and that it is *kami*'s work to quell it. In Japanese history, he notes, people have always prayed to *kami* for the calming of epidemics. *Kami*, as Koji Suga explains, should be understood as beings which possess extraordinary and unsurpassed abilities, and which are awesome and worthy of reverence no matter whether they are good or evil.

Turning to Sikhism, Teipaul Bainiwal adopts a fundamentally different view. The Sikh faith, he writes, teaches that everything happens according to *hukam* (Divine Order). Human beings may never be able to truly understand why these events occur because it is beyond our thinking and cannot be reduced to thought. Rather than attempting to explain Covid, the Sikh faith focuses on an internal journey cultivating true humility and being of service to others. In this context Nikky-Guninder Singh adds that Covid has reminded us of the interconnectedness of all things. We are all part of the vast living, breathing planetary organism. This realization radically shifts the view of human dominion over nature to one of partnership and kinship with nature combined with a commitment to justice for all beings.

In the Bahá'í chapter Wendi Momen confesses that she cannot determine whether the pandemic was sent by God to test humanity, or whether it is something humanity could have avoided by devoting our energies to operationalizing God's guidance. Or it may simply have been an accident. Yet she stresses that she learned one critical thing: it is one thing to read and meditate. But it is something quite different to act. Yet being and doing are two parts of life's work. George Merchant Ballentyne emphasizes this point. In response to suffering, he writes, Bahá'ís tend not to ask 'What kind of God would let this happen?' Instead they are more likely to ask what we can learn from the situation, how to use the experience as a stepping stone towards greater insight and better practice of our values and virtues.

Turning to Jainism, the prime theological focus has been on the human misuse of nature. As Vinod Kapashi explains, the imbalance in nature has been brought about by the ruthless quest for industrial development, the greedy exploitation of resources, the manipulation of natural harmony and the total disregard for animal sanctity. This is the context for understanding and confronting the Covid pandemic. According to Kumarpal Desai, Covid has underscored the imperative to treat nature with concern and respect. In this way it has united humanity in a common pursuit.

Nokuzula Mndende in the African chapter focuses on a different spiritual dimension. In confronting Covid, a central religious conviction is the belief that death does not mean the destruction of life. Rather it is a transition stage before an individual can enter the ancestral world. It is an opening into another sphere of existence. Hence though the individual has left this world, the deceased's spiritual body continues to function on another, higher plane. Hebron Ndlovu adds that, despite Covid's negative impact on normal life, it has not undermined African beliefs in ancestral veneration, mystical power, and the practice of rites of passage. He concludes that the indigenous worldviews, beliefs and values of the past still reign supreme in the hearts and minds of the African people.

For Zoroastrians Covid offers a different religious challenge. Jehangir Sarosh explains that the Ultimate in Zoroastrianism is Ahura Mazda, the Light of Wisdom that illuminates and sustains all that there is. In human beings it is the positive energy that enables good thoughts, words and actions. Ahura Mazda is not responsible for what happens in the material creation such as Covid. Rather such phenomena are due to the imbalance of natural forces. Each person, he writes, has the capacity to connect with the Light of Wisdom and thereby discover a remedy to bring things back into balance. In this context Koka Karishma emphasizes that the role of the human being in Zoroastrian belief is to increase the goodness in the world and remove negativity.

Feargus O'Connor in his Unitarianism chapter emphasizes that Covid raises serious theological questions. He asks: 'Why is such suffering tolerated by a supposedly just and loving religious dispensation?', and 'Can we really believe in an interventionist God?' Rejecting the concept of an omnipotent God who has limitless power, he endorses a form of process theism which he believes does not conflict with the facts of the cosmos as we presently apprehend them. Similarly, Jay Atkinson notes that, despite their theological diversity, most American UUs have humanistic and naturalistic leanings and would tend to reject any supernatural explanations of events, good or bad.

By contrast, Jolene Chu explains that Jehovah's Witnesses are united in believing that the world is experiencing the last days of human rulership. Appealing to Scripture, they expect the final days to be marked by war, lawlessness, famine, pestilence and fear. This is the context for understandings the Covid pandemic. Yet as Jehovah's Witnesses experience such tragic occurrences, they believe that divine relief is at hand. In this context Gary Perkins adds that Covid is a stark reminder to cherish our lives, using it to love God with our whole heart and mind, and to love our neighbours as ourselves.

Turning finally to Christian Science, Shirley Paulson asks: Where *is* God in the midst of a disease that threatens the whole world? Her answer is that there is a divine law of love that will always enable the world to thrive, operating even in the darkest hours of the pandemic. She insists that God never sent the darkness – rather God loves all of us enough to show us the way forward. Susan Searle echoes this view. A God that is all good, she writes, does not bring suffering upon creation. Hence illness – or any inharmony in our lives – should not be perceived as somehow inflicted by God. Covid, she argues, is not a punishment from God but an opportunity to grow spiritually.

It is clear from these different religious responses to Covid that there is no continuity of spiritual belief amongst religions. As we have seen, spiritual reality is conceived and understood in strikingly different ways. Yet despite these varied perspectives, contributors are united in their concern for humanity as a whole. Paradoxically, the Covid pandemic has demonstrated that the world is a global village. And it has awakened us to the need to care for all peoples across the globe.

31

What have we learned?

George D. Chryssides

When the British government imposed its lockdown, some of us were halfway through our ecumenical Lent groups at Lichfield Cathedral. During Lent, members of different denominations meet in groups of seven or eight to study and discuss a theme. The lockdown meant that everyone had to stay at home, although isolated individuals could form a 'bubble' with one exclusively designated household. When I suggested that our group might continue online, the response was, 'We don't think we know how to do that.' By the following year, online Lent groups were commonplace, and nearly everyone had managed to join one for the entire Lent course. Sunday services were streamed, with obvious benefits for the housebound, and could be replayed by anyone who did not quite catch part of the sermon or wanted to hear or see something again.

Several of our authors have highlighted how we have become more technologically savvy as a consequence of Covid, and how this has affected their arrangements for worship. They have also noted how the pandemic afforded opportunities to show acts of kindness, such as running errands for those who were shielding, and ensuring that the housebound – particularly those who lived alone – were all right.

Five questions

However, responding to Covid involves more than attending to such operational details. At the outset of our project, Dan Cohn-Sherbok and I formulated these five questions on which we suggested our contributors might comment.

How does your faith explain why such events occur?
How has it affected your religious practices?
What changes has it necessitated?
What differences might we expect once the pandemic is over?
What have we learned from it?

Our contributors have addressed these issues in varying degrees, since different faiths have required different responses. For some, the Covid pandemic has reinforced their theological beliefs, while for others it required serious doctrinal reflection. Some practices could readily be adapted to online versions, while others proved impossible, or encountered technological or theological difficulties. For example, while a funeral can be viewed online, there is inevitably a physical body to be laid to rest in the physical world. Key practices such as sacraments and initiation ceremonies presented problems: baptism, holy communion, *amrit* and *prasad* all require physical substances, raising the question of whether such rites should be suspended, or whether adaptation is possible. The Sikh *langar*, of course, is more than a mere custom, but often a necessary form of food provision, requiring the physical presence of food and people to serve it, raising the question, as one of our Sikh contributors pointed out, whether humanitarian work should take precedence over legal requirements. Another contributor mentioned online marriage (Chapter 8), which presents complicated legal problems as well as practical ones, if it is to avoid being a 'non-qualifying ceremony' – a particularly difficult issue if the couple are exchanging vows from different countries. The easing of lockdown restrictions has now caused people of faith to reflect on their adaptations, some reverting to traditional practices, while others perceive genuine benefits in some online adaptations, particularly those which enable the housebound to participate from their homes.

Religion or superstition?

The pandemic has also reminded us of humankind's frailty. *Homo sapiens* is the dominant species. The Jewish-Christian story of creation asserts that humankind has dominion over the whole of creation; yet notwithstanding our physical size and intelligence, we have been barely able to control a virus which can only be seen under a microscope. We have had to rely upon humanity's scientific expertise to reassert our status as the dominant species.

However, not everyone has wanted to rely on science, and one downside of the pandemic was that it unleashed a horde of conspiracy theories, counterfeit cures and quack remedies. Even the US President Donald Trump entertained the idea that ingesting bleach might be solution (BBC 2020). For the most part, the various religions that have featured in this volume have favoured scientific advance, and many of us have made our religious buildings available for vaccination clinics, and encouraged members to protect themselves. On the more negative side, it is regrettable that some religious believers have perceived their faith as an alternative to science. Some 22 per cent of white evangelical Christians in the United States have been opposed to vaccination, claiming biblical support for the belief that unaided divine protection would give them immunity from the virus. For a number of religious adherents, the objections have been quasi-scientific. Some have believed that the vaccines were developed too quickly, with insufficient testing. For others, there was a concern about the ingredients. It was rumoured in certain circles that the vaccines contained aborted foetal cells – a claim which, if true, would be abhorrent to pro-life advocates. Others believed that there were porcine or bovine ingredients in the vaccines, which would have been offensive to Muslims and Hindus.

The rumour about human foetuses was false, although in past generations foetal tissue was used in the testing of drugs and vaccines (Nebraska Medicine 2021). The Vatican has stated that vaccination is morally acceptable, and indeed desirable. Pfizer, Moderna and AstraZeneca, evidently, do not contain porcine or bovine gelatine, although some other companies do not declare their ingredients. Muslims appear to be divided on the issue of whether porcine ingredients would be acceptable: in 2020 the United Arab Emirates' Fatwa Council expressed the opinion that they would be halal if chemically treated, but other Islamic authorities have disagreed. Of course, such concerns do not merit an anti-vaxx stance, but careful discrimination about the vaccine one accepts.

In other circles – mainly in the US Protestant evangelical tradition – the objection to vaccination has been theological: one should trust in God rather than humanity for protection against the virus. Proponents of this position typically emphasize miraculous healing, and God's design of the human body with the ability to heal itself. Televangelist Kenneth Copeland, in a broadcast during the pandemic, blew into the camera, claiming that he was conveying the wind of God, which would dispel the virus that was caused by Satan, and that it would now be gone for ever (Woodward 2020). T.N.T. Ministries continues to offer T-shirts for sale, bearing the slogan, 'Fully vaccinated by the blood of Jesus,' available in six different sizes (T.N.T. Ministries 2022). (T.N.T. stands for 'Teaching New Testament', but also alludes to the explosive trinitrotoluene, signifying the Gospel's power.) Another Christian fundamentalist, David Eelles, who founded Unleavened Bread Ministries, has authored a book entitled *God's Vaccine*, which copiously quotes the Bible's assurance of divine protection, placing great emphasis on Psalm 91: 'There shall no evil befall thee, neither shall any plague come nigh thy dwelling.' Of course it should not be thought that all Christian fundamentalists adopt this position, and many conservative Christian leaders have disagreed strongly. Franklin Graham contended that Jesus would have advocated vaccination, and Pastor Robert Jeffress argued that, just as life inside the womb was a gift from God, so was life outside it, and should be protected by vaccine. J. D. Greer, the President of the Southern Baptist Church, allowed himself to be photographed being vaccinated, and tweeted the picture (Brigham 2021).

Many readers will be familiar with the story of the pious man who refused offers of rescue when trapped in his house amid rising flood water. Helpers variously sent him a life belt, a boat and a helicopter. (There are variants of the story.) Each time, he declined, insisting that God would rescue him. Finally, he died, submerged in the flood water. On arrival at the pearly gates, he asked God why he did not come to his rescue, to which God replied, 'I sent you a life belt, a boat, and a helicopter. What more did you want from me?' The import of the story, of course, is the old adage, 'God helps those who help themselves,' meaning that we should not expect divine intervention as a substitute for the use of human initiative. To do so is to cross the boundary between religion and superstition.

Why do pandemics happen?

The first of our five questions is no doubt the most difficult. Vast tomes have been written on the problem of evil throughout the centuries, and none of our contributors claim to have resolved an issue of such magnitude within their allocated wordage. At the risk of appearing to solve a centuries-old problem, however, I should like to conclude this anthology by making a few observations on the question. We might well agree that the pandemic should not be viewed as divine punishment. Although the Jewish-Christian Bible appears to portray God as rewarding his people for being righteous, and punishing them for their disobedience, such an explanation seems implausible. Good and evil people alike have equally suffered from the pandemic, the saintly no less than the sinful. Jesus once referred to another disaster with which his hearers would have been familiar – a tower in Siloam which collapsed. He asked, 'Do you think they were more guilty than all the others living in Jerusalem? I tell you, no!' (Lk. 13.4-5). However, he added, 'But unless you repent, you too will all perish.'

Jesus was suggesting that, although disaster is not related to sin on a one-to-one basis, nonetheless there is a connection between human behaviour and human suffering. One or two contributors pointed out that, whether pandemic was due to unhygienic conditions in a Wuhan meat market, or to a laboratory accident in the Wuhan Institute of Virology, human behaviour was responsible, even if unintentional. As a vegetarian, I might be tempted to feel virtuous, since there would be no meat markets if everyone, like myself, lived on plant-based products. However, many scientists believe that the cause of pandemics goes wider. For example, deforestation has forced animals to leave their forest dwellings, thus causing them to come into greater contact with humans, and increasing the risk of viruses jumping species – a phenomenon known as 'zoonotic spillover' (Stand For Trees 2022).

Historically, the free will defence has not proved popular among philosophers and theologians as a solution to the problem of evil, the main objection being that it does not account for natural disasters. However, it may have more mileage than is commonly supposed, as we are becoming increasingly aware that the boundaries between natural and human events are blurred. Climate change, global warming, famine, disease and of course pandemics have substantial human causes.

Some of us have made adjustments to our lifestyle, working at home, holding online meetings instead of travelling long distances and making fewer journeys. However, in the first four months of 2020, there was a 55 per cent rise in rainforest destruction in Brazil, losing 464 square miles of trees – only one example of the way in which humankind is destroying its environment (Brown 2020). In the UK, as soon as lockdown restrictions were sufficiently lifted to allow foreign travel, tourists rushed off to Spain and Portugal, increasing their carbon footprint by air travel, and subsequently complaining about airport congestion and tour companies that left them stranded abroad. While the pandemic was still raging, Vladimir Putin started a war in Ukraine, causing mass death and destruction, resulting in around seven million Ukrainians fleeing their home country, and a similar number internally displaced.

Nations spend billions of dollars on military expenditure: in June 2022 it was reported that the United States had contributed $56 billion dollars in weapons to the war in Ukraine alone (CNBC 2022). In the United Kingdom alone the cost of crime is at least £50 billion, perhaps as much as £100 billion a year. Just imagine what could be achieved if those monies were channelled into medical research, healthcare, environmental protection and education instead! Perhaps we would not achieve a perfect world, but we could undoubtedly reduce the amount of sickness and suffering on earth, and find ways of eliminating diseases that have caused so much misery and death. The word 'sin', used in Christian and Jewish theology, is unpopular in common parlance, but it is a salutary exercise to look at the daily news reports in the media and reflect on the number of items in which human sin has some bearing.

It is sometimes remarked that a pandemic like the one we are continuing to experience is a great leveller, since it can affect anyone from a beggar to a monarch. In the UK it claimed victims in high government office, and members of the royal family. However, it would be wrong to infer that the virus has somehow made everyone equal. This is not the case: some people have mild symptoms, while others suffer from 'long Covid'; some recover rapidly, while others die. Countries with high-density population, crowded living conditions and poor sanitation have inevitably proved to be much more prone to the virus than those with greater wealth and better medical provision. It has been noted that those who belong to Black, Asian and Minority Ethnic communities have been at greater risk of catching the virus. Evidently, this is not due to genetic characteristics, but rather that they are more likely to have poorer living conditions, or to have jobs that bring them into contact with many more people, for example, taxi drivers, shop assistants or factory workers. These inequalities are of human creation, exacerbated by racism and discrimination. Christians frequently quote Paul's assertion that 'There is neither Jew nor Gentile, neither slave nor free, nor is there male and female, for you are all one in Christ Jesus' (Gal. 3.28). Sadly, we are far from reaching this ideal.

How long might it take for human beings to bring the earth to a satisfactory state? Religions typically place humankind in the earth's last days. This is no doubt because the human race could swiftly be brought to an end, whether through a nuclear holocaust, meteoric impact or another even more serious pandemic, or – as some religions have suggested – through supernatural intervention, for example, a final battle such as Armageddon. However, without such possibilities, scientists have estimated that the planet earth could sustain life for as much as one billion, or even 1.5 billion years, if appropriately managed. If this is correct, then perhaps humankind is somewhere near the beginning. If our resolve and resources are channelled correctly, with the help of our various religious teachings, perhaps humanity has a future – but we have a long way to go.

References

BBC. (2020). 'Coronavirus: Outcry after Trump Suggests Injecting Disinfectant as Treatment'. 24 April. Accessible online at URL: www.bbc.co.uk/news/world-us-canada-52407177.

Brigham, Bob. (2021). 'White Evangelical Resistance Is Obstacle in Vaccination Effort'. *New York Times*. 7 October. Accessible online at URL: www.nytimes.com/2021/04/05/us/covid-vaccine-evangelicals.html.

Brown, Kimberley. (2020). 'The Hidden Toll of Lockdown on Rainforests'. *BBC Future*. 19 May. Accessible online at URL: www.bbc.com/future/article/20200518-why-lockdown-is-harming-the-amazon-rainforest.

Joi, Priya. (2020). '10 Things We Have Now Learned about COVID-19'. *VaccinesWork*. 8 October. Accessible online at URL: www.gavi.org/vaccineswork/10-things-we-have-now-learned-about-covid-19?gclid=EAIaIQobChMI6d344Kqm-glVRrDtCh33zgbQEAAYASAAEgItA_D_BwE.

Macias, Amanda. (2022). 'Here's a Look at the $5.6 Billion in Firepower the U.S. Has Committed to Ukraine in Its Fight against Russia'. *CNBC*. 17 June. Accessible online at URL: www.cnbc.com/2022/06/17/russia-ukraine-war-summary-of-weapons-us-has-given-to-ukraine.html.

Nebraska Medicine. (2021). 'You Asked, We Answered: Do the COVID-19 Vaccines Contain Aborted Fetal Cells?' www.nebraskamed.com/COVID/you-asked-we-answered-do-the-covid-19-vaccines-contain-aborted-fetal-cells.

Stand for Trees. (2022). 'Deforestation and Covid-19: Nature Bites Back'. https://standfortrees.org/blog/deforestation-covid/.

T.N.T. Ministries. (2022). Online Bookstore. Accessible online at URL: www.tntministriesonline.org.

Woodward, Alex. (2020). 'Coronavirus: Televangelist Kenneth Copeland 'Blows Wind of God' at Covid-19 to 'Destroy' Pandemic'. *The Independent*. 6 April. Accessible online at URL: https://www.independent.co.uk/news/world/americas/kenneth-copeland-blow-coronavirus-pray-sermon-trump-televangelist-a9448561.html.

Index